Parkinson's Disease

A Comprehensive Guide How to Treat Parkinson Disease

(Understanding the Disease Managing Your Symptoms and Navigating Treatment)

Jason Grimm

Published By **Andrew Zen**

Jason Grimm

All Rights Reserved

Parkinson's Disease: A Comprehensive Guide How to Treat Parkinson Disease (Understanding the Disease Managing Your Symptoms and Navigating Treatment)

ISBN 978-0-9938088-7-6

Legal & Disclaimer

Table Of Contents

Chapter 1: It's Always A Good Time To Start Exercising (But The Sooner The Better) 1

Chapter 2: Challenging You To Change Yourself.. 5

Chapter 3: Target And Reduce Your Symptoms With Specific Exercises 12

Chapter 4: Use Your Buddies, Space And Activities To Stay Motivated 29

Chapter 5: Exercising Your Mind Is As Important As Exercising Your Body 37

Chapter 6: What Exactly Is Parkinson's Disease?... 50

Chapter 7: Who Is At Risk For Parkinson's Disease?... 55

Chapter 8: What Is The Specific Of What My Doctor Will Look At? 63

Chapter 9: Tips For Living Well With Parkinson's... 74

Chapter 10: Therapy Based On Movement 80

Chapter 11: Parkinson's Disease 86

Chapter 12: Non-Movement Symptoms 93

Chapter 13: How Is It Treated? 103

Chapter 14: What's The Outlook Of Parkinson's Disease? 113

Chapter 15: What To Know About Parkinson's Diet 127

Chapter 16: Antioxidant-Containing Foods 134

Chapter 17: Parkinson's Disease Natural Treatments 143

Chapter 18: The Parkinson's Disease: What Is It? 155

Chapter 19: Where Does It Come From? 157

Chapter 20: What Signs Should I Look For? 162

Chapter 21: The Parkinson's Disease Progression 167

Chapter 22: Complications 172

Chapter 23: Is There A Cure, And If So, What Treatment Options Are Available? 177

Chapter 1: It's Always A Good Time To Start Exercising (But The Sooner The Better)

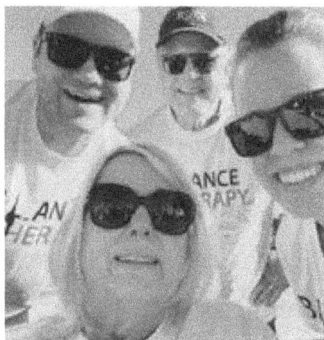

You might be not familiar with exercise, or are you are out of the habit. You may be exercising but not for the purpose of PD. Research shows that those suffering from Parkinson's disease have already been withdrawn from activities like leisure, sports or recreation activities by the time the diagnosis.

The general trend of a more relaxed life style, coupled with the progressive loss of spatial and body awareness, which is a hallmark of PD causes difficulties in self-monitoring. This makes it difficult to correct minor or slow movements, as well as tilted postures.

Exercise can be a powerful way to reset neural connections within the brain, allowing moving simpler. Maintaining PD-specific principles that are good is essential.

Technically speaking, the earlier you can begin to exercise following diagnosis it is the better. Early exercisers safeguard the dopamine neurons present and help keep their. Additionally, exercise can make impaired dopamine systems work better. The early exercise can also increase the amount of dopamine receptors inside the brain. In simple terms, the brain absorbs any dopamine more efficiently and quicker. The result is in fewer signs.

It's not too late to begin working out. People who exercise later also benefit from their regimen of exercise, however it is more time-consuming to achieve the results. Therefore, if you are starting earlier in the progression of Parkinson's Be patient while you adjust to this change in your lifestyle.

Additionally, the mental health of people who begin exercising later to people who do any exercise is improved due to less inflammation greater blood flow to the brain and better functioning the brain's circuits. Be aware that healthy brains have the capacity to battle PD and also exercise helps to maintain a healthy brain regardless of time.

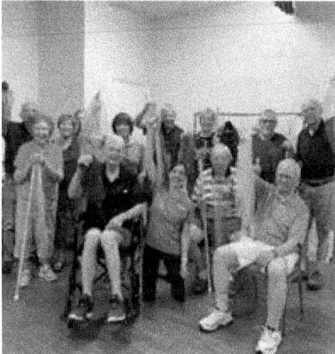

Whatever your position on your journey to defeat PD it is the main factor is to get going now, while you're contemplating the issue. If you're not sure how to begin, you can choose the right form or movement of exercise that you'll be able to do to make it harder.

When you begin working out, keep going! This is a lifetime commitment to keep your body and brain operating at their best to the maximum extent possible.

Chapter 2: Challenging You To Change Yourself

Have you heard of the phrase "If it isn't challenging you, it isn't changing you"? Your goal for your workout programme should be changing your brain, as that's what will reduce PD symptoms.

Animal studies show that exercising is the sole thing we aware of that could slow the progress of PD. If you'd like to boost your PD overall health, then a specific exercise regimen that targets PD and has a long and short-term focused on goals is suggested. It requires structure, planning and repetition however, you are able to do it.

A rigorous exercise regimen is the best way to alter the neural wiring of your brain so that you can move more easily. It's all about pushing over your own self-determined speed, intensity, and movement range. This is basically playing until you master the appear to be a good idea.

It is here that it is that magic happens to patients with Parkinson's disease. If you feel that the movement isn't natural at first, then you're most likely performing the right thing. Your goal is to the exercise routine to stimulate the brain's attention and then change it's wiring by repeating the exercise repeatedly.

You may think you're taking excessive measures, however being able to perform your movements with vigor and intent is essential for the brain to develop new abilities and keep the ability to move. Particularly, if you are looking to alter the wiring that your brain uses to facilitate better movements, you should challenge you in two zones: cardio exercise and exercise that is functional.

What are you able to do if you're not "exercising" per se? Scream and squeak is what. It's good to exercise your muscles for people suffering from Parkinson's. We'll hear this from an experienced PwP Chrystal Kafka.

Pearls made from PwP

"It's vital to stay in motion, not merely an hour of intense workout, then lay down for all day, or, if like me, all every day! If you're preparing to be an accomplished concert pianist you must be in a hurry and with purpose throughout our working day as is possible. That is, move about with enthusiasm in the time you're not working out.

Simply put, raising the heart rate by aerobic exercise improves the blood flow to the brain. In boosting the circulation of the brain, you're increasing the amount of work memory and attention areas that are involved in understanding or recalling what normal motion feels like.

Each movement that is functional is accompanied by a specific pathway of neurons that are located in the brain. In the case of PD and PD, the previous neural pathways to movements are dying. The time is now to safeguard those remaining neural pathways and create new ones that can be used for moving. This is accomplished by stimulating the brain through aerobic exercise, followed by the practice of moves that are intense and hard.

Pearls taken from a PwP

"In my PD experience, I've encountered problems with autonomic or conscious coordination. Exercise aids muscles and nerves to be reorganized and better communicate throughout every movement.- Chrystal Kafka

What is the ideal amount of time you should be exercising, you might ask?

An easy way to gauge the intensity of your work is to test your capacity to speak while working out. It will be clear that you're at a high level of productivity when you are able to speak in short phrases.

Particularly, talk to your physical therapist, trainer to assist you in calculating your heart rate goal and then invest in an electronic heart rate monitor.

Exercise Rx research conducted by Cleveland Clinic. Cleveland Clinic showed a 35 percent reduction in the symptoms of just cycling with a speedy pace at a maximum of 80-90 rotations per minute, for 45-60 mins.

Pearls derived from a PwP

"Exercise when you are at the top in your PD medication or when the medications are "ON" for greater brain activity. Also, it improves your movement precision as well as freedom of movements."

Go BIG and Fast to Keep Your Skills Up

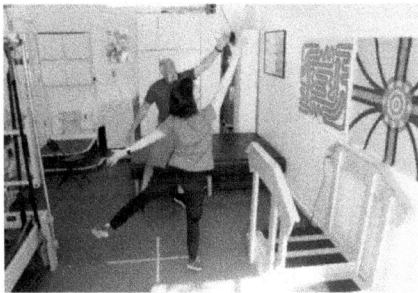

Are you still with me? You're doing well, because things are getting really exciting.

Training in skills allows you to execute meaningful actions with more ease, like changing bed positions as well as getting into and out of chairs, walking and changing direction when walking.

The functional movements described above are ones which become harder in the course of PD. The goal is to learn what the normal motion feels and feels like throughout your daily life.

The key is having a body that is flexible capable of shifting the weight in a safe manner and knowing the best way to go going to be the best, and making sure you are practicing with the maximum amount of efforts!

Exercises that help improve your capabilities are actually just an improved version of your everyday routine moves. As with Parkinson's it is essential to learn those movements you wish to maintain. That may mean another set of eyes and an example from a trained expert such as a Parkinson's specific trainer or physical therapy.

Exercise Rx: When you have a grasp on the strength of your movements then you must practice them with a lot of effort. If you are practicing the Parkinson's particular motion, you should aim for distinct endings and beginnings, as you move between extremes to next. The sequences of movements should feel like a ball, but they will be clearly defined.

Let's take "BIG walking" as an illustration. You may have heard about Lee Silverman Voice Therapy (LSVT) BIG(r) or LSVT LOUD(r) treatment. In recent times, a new variation of BIG therapy came to be known as PWR! Moves(r). They were both developed by the same scientist, Becky Farley, PT, PhD.

Chapter 3: Target And Reduce Your Symptoms With Specific Exercises

The most exciting benefits of exercising is the fact that it helps reduce symptoms. The key is to pick the right exercises to address specific symptoms. Each of these signs can be effectively addressed through an educated training program specifically designed for people with PD.

Common symptoms of motor dysfunction include:

* Tightness of the spine and stiffness of the trunk.

* It is difficult to shift weight

* Minor moves

* Slow motions

* Tucked into a position

* Difficulty in changing position

It is difficult to change directions when walking

* Freezing

* Impairment of body and spatial perception

* Inadequate movement timing

* It is difficult to do two different things simultaneously

Exercise according to your PD symptoms is a constantly evolving both physically and mentally. It will require you to be a bit more challenging, and learning more about your body during the years and months ahead. Certain activities are likely to benefit your body differently than others, according to your personality, the days, medications as well as your water intake as well as your sleep quality eating, mood etc. PD symptoms differ greatly between individuals. Certain kinds of exercises may be more beneficial for your body, but not for other.

Easing Stiffness

The rigidity of the spine makes it hard to be able to move.

Training Rx: Concentrate on exercises which stretch your spine into and out of side bends, twists and forward flexion as well as backward extension. The yoga, the BIG Therapy PD Warrior and PWR!Moves are great examples of exercises that assist in improving the flexibility of the spine. Move from one end to the next and repeat 20 times per day. You should stretch beyond your own limit of motion. It should feel like you are stretching!

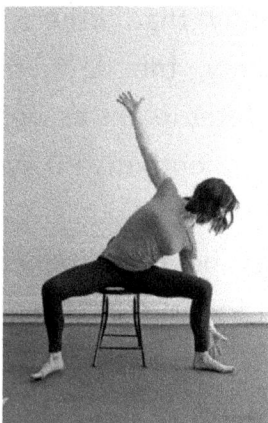

The exercise prescription Yoga can be an excellent outlet to release the rigidity. You should focus upon "flow," i.e. moving

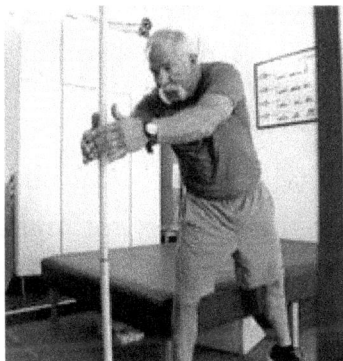

between poses frequently instead of holding poses all the duration. Make sure you are fully at the entire range of motion within each posture before moving on to the next.

Exercise Rx: Research indicates that intense cycling decreases stiffness and tremors in the PwP. While it's not "stretching," it still assists. It's best to do an 80-90 rpm every minute for a period of 45 minutes.

Improving Weight Shifting and Small Movements

The difficulty of shifting weight is another sign that may be present for people suffering from Parkinson's disease. The movement process is not possible without the ability to shift weight. Basic movements, like walking require shifts in weight.

It is logical that walking could be challenging in the event that you're not unloading your leg sufficiently to allow your other leg. While walking, you are expected to shift between one foot and another. In PD it is less likely that weight shifting occurs and causes a significant amount of duration walking with both feet on the ground when walking. The tiny, unshuffled or strenuous steps draw the body of vitality in the course of walking.

Exercise Rx: Do big, intense moves. You'll feel as if you're rocking between two sides and

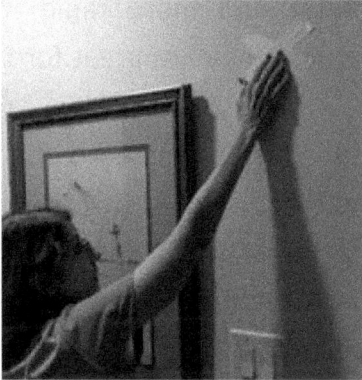

moving shifting from side to side between extremes towards the opposite in a regular manner for big weight shifts. You can also add arm movements to a target from every direction, to ensure you stay in the right direction. This can be done in a sitting position or standing.

Yoga, PWR!Moves, and LSVT BIG Therapy are a good example of this.

Improving Slow Movements

The slowness of your movements is a major problem for people who suffer from PD. The character of the disease strips the person of their ability to assess the how you move and hinders your ability to judge how well you're doing. Greater and more rapid moves are harder however they are great for those with Parkinson's disease. Utilizing resistance, targets and effert to increase the speed of movements. Achieving body awareness is essential factor in people suffering from PD and creating a feedback mechanism can make a difference.

Exercise Rx: Perform more intense exercises. Fast and small moves are not enough of a challenge for people with PwP. Make every effort to provoke larger and faster moves and set up an effective feedback mechanism that keeps your movements within control.

Training Rx for Exercise: Do higher effort exercises using the treadmill. The treadmill is great for those with PwP because they stop your body from automatically selecting a slow speed as you go along. Pick a incline or speed that's more challenging and fast than what you'd like, and then go for the treadmill for about 45 minutes. After that then you've completed your cardio and fitness training to the end of the day.

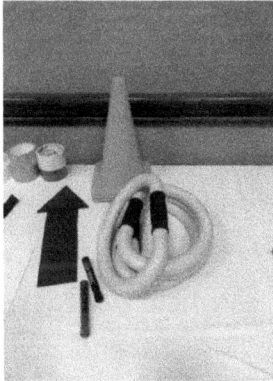

Training intervals is another great method to train as you build up your endurance. Simply walk around on a treadmill for 30 seconds to three minutes per minute. It's an excellent method to gain the amount of repetitions and intensities you require.

Using Feedback Mechanisms to Improve Body and Spatial Awareness

The body and spatial awareness slips off so gradually in those who suffer from PD and PD that it may be overlooked until it develops into an issue. In this chapter you'll learn build feedback mechanisms to help you stay aware of your movement quality.

If you really want to remain independent for as long as you can, you must seek out guidance and feedback from a professional initially and then maintain this throughout the process. This can help you determine which opportunities exist to enhance and sustain your capabilities. If you're not equipped with additional eyes, one option is to create environmental signals that will guide you to specific movements.

Exercise Rx: Draw an area on the wall or floor by using tape. You can reach it each period of time. You may need to increase the effort you exert through slapping, hitting, and kicking the targets in order to increase the speed and size of your moves. Boxing classes designed for PD can be a perfect illustration of this. The addition of jumps and resistance are another method to create the effort.

Video can also be a great method of feedback.

Exercise Rx: Take an image of you moving through the motions, and you'll know exactly what I'm talking about. You may think your movements are "normal," but watching the video replays will reveal the true nature of your tendency to slow, slump or sluggish.

Mirrors, however, aren't the best source of feedback in the form of images. The brain can only perceive the things it is conditioned to see If you only rely on mirrors for feedback. A replaying of your own doing something is far more beneficial.

Exercise Rx Smovey vibroswings, hand held rings fitted with ball bearings which aid many suffering from Parkinson's during their workouts. The resonant vibrations created by the ball bearings spinning while the rings are swung may induce a feeling of relaxation, renewal as well as body awareness. When you move them they create an emitted sound as well as a vibrating sensation. This is an excellent source of audio as well as tactile feedback. It is possible to walk around with them or practice Smovey-related exercises using YouTube video or DVDs. It is my suggestion to explore them and see which

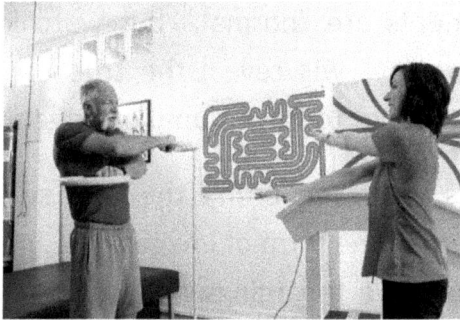

ones are right for you.

Keeping It Snappy

Timing of movements is vital, however it changes with the progress of PD. All day activities such as moving your arms and walking need an inner sense of time. So, adding rhythmic signals like metronomes or music could ensure that your body is in sync.

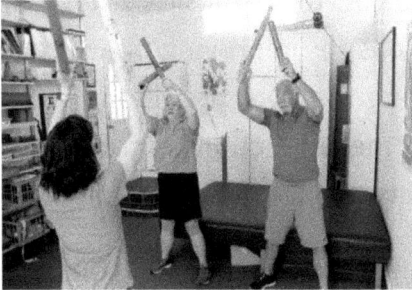

Your brain's response will be better when you tap on its reward centers while doing movements that are rhythmic. The preferred music you listen to is a good option because it triggers the brain with a positive emotion and increase the amount of dopamine released by the brain. It makes the movement feel more natural and pleasurable.

Be aware of the magnitude of your movements whenever you use the rhythmic cues. It isn't a good idea to compromise the dimensions of your moves so that you can keep pace with the beat.

The brain is more willing to adapt if you feel satisfied and happy while doing and moving, so pick a beat or a tune you like. The research has shown that music plays significant implications for improving understanding and modulating the your attention. The ability to optimize these functions is crucial for anyone who wants to alter the way you think.

It is important for your workouts to be challenging but doable. Begin with a more gradual but still demanding beat before speeding to a higher level in time through practice. Remember to think "big and timely," not "small and timely," even if it is necessary to begin at an earlier pace.

If you're using a smartphone, phone, consider using metronome.com, the Metronome Pro app and a set of earbudsand you'll be carrying the metronome on you whenever you travel. Also, there are metronome wristbands as well as other devices for wear that beat in rhythm. So, you'll marches in sync with the beat of a drum that is more stable as opposed to the drum that you have in your headand without having anyone else know.

Improving Posture

The ability to maintain a tall posture versus a smaller one isn't as easy to do to help people with PwP. The upright posture may be slowly, but steadily, slipping by the side of the road if you're not conscious and attentive.

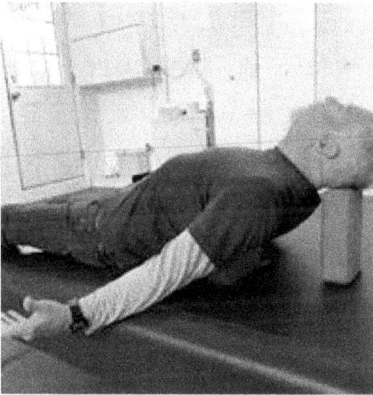

The reason for this is that, when you suffer from PD muscle groups in your back which support you against gravity weaken and weak. In addition, the muscles at the front are overly active and tight which results in, guess the answer, a higher stooped posture. The way that posture is impaired influences many areas of motion.

Pearl of a PwP

"We are unable to see what "up" is located in the space. Do a lot of squeezes on your glutes and your core whenever you're in a position to stand around."-Chrystal Kafka

The muscles that are tight in front as well as weak muscles in the back make your shoulders, head as well as your chest and the trunk to a forward posture. This is important since this bending posture moves your weight to the feet in front while standing or walking. It's hard to take large enough steps with your hips... in the behind. As time passes, your brain starts to assume that your slumped posture is actually straight. It also increases the likelihood of falling down as well as freezing PwP.

Training Rx for Exercise: to strengthen and preserve upright posture move and stretch the muscles that are located in front part of the body. This will also increase the strength and power of those muscles located in the back. By lifting and reaching your legs and arms while lying on your stomach or sitting with your elbows can be the best way to do this. Imagine straight leg raises or bent leg raises, snow angels and superman movements from your stomach or supported

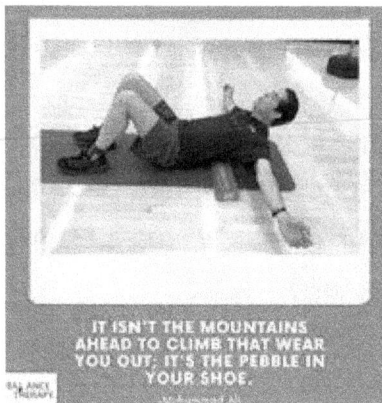

IT ISN'T THE MOUNTAINS AHEAD TO CLIMB THAT WEAR YOU OUT; IT'S THE PEBBLE IN YOUR SHOE.

with your elbows.

It is also beneficial to lay down on your back and place your body on a stand, with your head and shoulders secured by a wall stretching your neck and lengthening it while lifting the arm to the side. The abrasive support of the surfaces helps to maintain posture and activates the postural muscles as you move.

For physical therapy, such as in physical therapy, I'll put the sandbag, which weighs 15 pounds, inside a backpack, and then have my patients strap it to the body's front. It causes their upright postural muscles to work in walking and standing. This serves as a great reminding of how inactive the muscles will be if you're not paying attention. It is important to note that this exercise may not work for everyone suffering from PD So, make sure to consult your doctor, PT or a trainer prior to attempting this.

Chapter 4: Use Your Buddies, Space And Activities To Stay Motivated

The exercise routine you've chosen is designed to keep you energized, aware and able into the future. To achieve this you have to keep doing your routine consistently and have a clear goal all the way to that future. For that it is essential to remain active in your pursuits and motivate yourself to do the same level. As per Sarah King, PT, DPT "Make it fun, social, and accountable."

Apart from being mindful of the improvement

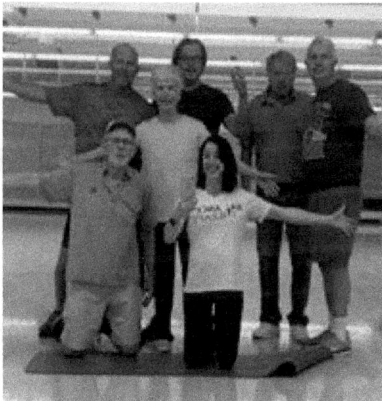

in the motor and brain skills which exercise can bring there are other efficient ways to motivate yourself to adhere to your workout regimen.

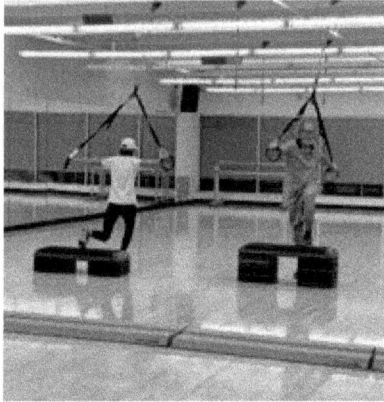

Bring a Friend Along

The brain is stimulated whenever the exercise can be viewed as emotionally satisfying. Take your exercise routine as an occasion to work with your fellow athletes.

It has been discovered that loneliness can accelerate the progress of Parkinson's disease. The other factors are the lack of sleep, poverty or exercise. In these cases it is possible to tackle your sedentary lifestyle by working out more and involvement in other activities.

When you are doing this in a communal, social environment, you will be able to enrich your social circle, make relationships and be a positive influence to the wider community. Additionally, it will help in reducing the speed of PD progress.

Pearl of a PwP

"Exercising on your own can be lonely. There's no reason to feel the only one fighting Parkinson's. Additionally, your brain is given an increase when your activity is exciting, thrilling and also social. In addition, exercise buddies motivate and inspire to push you. This is an incredible phenomenon is certain to have seen, and it's too crucial to overlook.

Engaging in exercise with your friends can make an ideal environment for less self-deprecation and increased camaraderie and friendship. There are limitations that we all face in some form or the other." The author is Chrystal Kafka

Try setting the time for sessions with a specific instructor for PD as part of your fitness routine. Exercise classes are a excellent way to exercise within the company of your peers as well as your mentors. The exercise routine you choose to take part in should be like a party and not as a solo exercise routine.

This is why the idea of doing fitness at home on your own might not be the ideal option for those suffering from PD. If you are forced to do it, or you just want working out on your own There are a variety of wonderful internet-based programs that include online communities, as well as applications for smart phones that are designed specifically for those who suffer from PD.

Bring A Furry Friend Along

They are a great walking companion They can also be very cuddly, and are great conversation starters in the neighborhood. It is recommended to get the most well-trained pet or trainer for your dog. You should take special care when you own a dog as well as PD or PD, and want your bond with your pet to be as relaxing and satisfying as it can be.

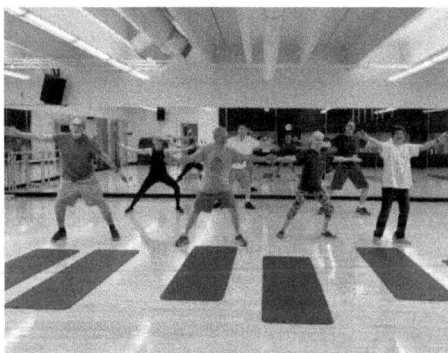

Create Your Perfect Space

As well as creating camaraderie in your workout you can also create your environment in a more enriching way. Take note of where you're and with whom you're during your workout, since the appropriate environment has been proven to encourage positive brain change. The goal is to make it seem like an unforgettable and interactive moment. Exercise, for instance, in nature is a great opportunity to activate the reward centers in your brain.

Another way to improve the ambience of your home is by adding pleasing sound, lighting or music. So, be kind to yourself! Your brain will appreciate it.

Engage in Creative, Meaningful and Motivating Movements

Your brain is more likely to make positive changes when the task has meaning, creativity as well as adventurous. It is here that novel experiences are a major factor.

Recreational activities such as sports or planned exercises, as well as group exercise classes that are based on community should be included in your daily routine. Additionally "exergaming" is a fun alternative that you can try and fall in love with. (See this list of resources)

Set goals and an element of fun will stimulate your brain, too.

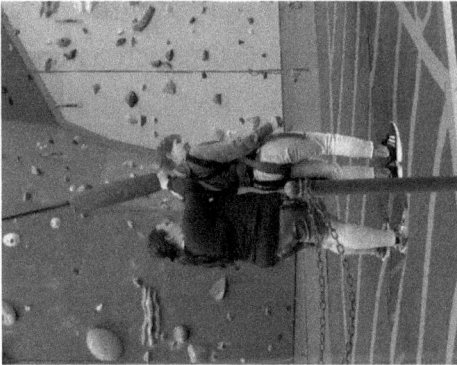

Explore and think outside of your comfort zone if you're looking to keep your mind and body working in a better way. Make sure to maintain your sense of humor intact and take a step back in stepping outside your familiar area. Being open-minded is essential in order to live the fullest life possible as a person with PD.

Pearls taken from PwP

"I keep going because I still find it interesting." Paul Nitze

Find out how someone with Parkinson's can keep life and PDfascinating with a myriad of physical and mental tasks such as continuous learning, challenging tasks, helping others, taking part in a social setting as well as a variety of exercise options, all while maintaining an active life style. The PWP is working to maintain cognition, motor and social performance through regular usage for WII Balance games, Musical Chairs (home-made vibro-acoustic therapies] as well as recumbent bicycles Boxing, various kinds of exercises, rehabilitation, audio-visual entrainment (AVE) as well as neuro-feedback. high-intensity work, wearable monitoring equipment, PD education, standard PD medicines, as well as old-fashioned playing around. The activities and actions have an impact on autonomic functioning such as tiredness, sleep, mood as well as interactions with others." Dan Novak

Chapter 5: Exercising Your Mind Is As Important As Exercising Your Body

In earlier sections, we've talked about strategies to test your body to alter your brain's structure and also strategies to keep yourself focused to follow your regimen to reap the maximum benefits. This time, we'll discuss how you can test and strengthen your brain in order to be able to multitask, stay balanced and perform your movements with

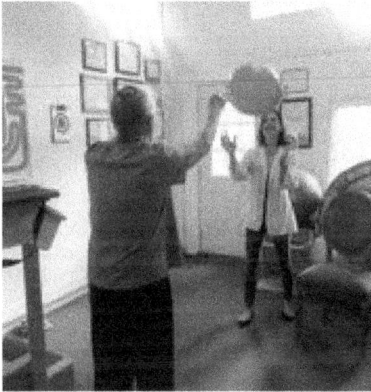

ease.

Thinking and Moving Simultaneously

The ability to perform two things simultaneously is a valuable capability that could begin to fall off in the early phases of PD. A lot of things that we like the most call for dual-tasking or performing multiple activities at the same time.

Dual-tasking can be a challenge for PwP as they are required to consider routine movements that used to be routine, such as the swing of arms while walking like. If PwP embark on a seemingly easy walk with a deliberate activity like talking or listening to music, their balance, posture security, and the quality of movements can be affected.

You may be able to talk when walking but the steps start to get shuffled and your arms move less because of. The thought process can interfere with the movements of your body. In addition, straining your muscles like that drains your energy, leads to fatigue, and can increase the likelihood of falling.

Dual-tasking could be improved through practice and exercises. Exercise your mind is the same as exercising your body, and you'll be working out regardless (because you're amazing!) make sure to keep it going with mentally challenging games, exercises that help build awareness of the environment as well as other activities.

The ever-changing technology has proven to be a fantastic way to engage in physical and cognitive training through PwP. There are many options in my list of resources and encourage you to look it up. For now, let me offer my next exercise regimen.

exercise Rx: If are using a smart phone and want to install Clock Yourself. Clock Yourself app. It's a great tool for practicing the art of doing your thinking. This application combines mental and physical exercise to help you practice the art of reactive stepping. It will also meet you at the place you are by providing numerous levels of intensity in a progressive manner.

Exercises that can be used to dual-task are counting backwards by threes, uttering all the words you can in just a few minutes and choosing a topic for example, such as things you can find at the beach or inside the refrigerator, and then sort them alphabetically.

So long as you're in a safe place and you aren't texting when driving, you won't be at risk of losing. In addition, by increasing your physical and mental effort that you put into your scheduled PD program it will help you save energy and time in the day.

If you're having issues in your balance or security you must work with an PD trainer at the beginning in order to track the movements of your body and assist you in directing your thinking process in the right direction.

In addition to thinking-related tasks security, the quality of movements and posture are the most important factors. If one of these is at risk, you should reduce your thinking tasks until you're ready into more difficult cognitive tasks.

Training Rx. If worry about your balance or slipping, get started by riding a stationary bicycle. add mental work starting there. If you and your friend find your dominant mind dominating, as in reduce or eliminate your thinking tasks for the moment.

Being able to carry conversations that are meaningful during the course of a normal walk is a problem with quality of life for people with PwP, a second option to consider, should it be appropriate, is walking with a friend.

Talking and moving is a typical symptom of people with PwP. Thus, simply by speaking and walking with a friend, you're creating the conditions for your PD brain for success through the following actions:

• Keeping it enjoyable and entertaining

* Keep it fun and social

* Controlling your breathing as well as practicing with your voice

• Getting feedback from a partner regarding your movement quality as well as your voice, posture, and your safety

• Organizing your thoughts, and flow of communication

If you think the task is like it's so tedious or demanding that you're not even interested in exercising then choose a more exciting activity like throwing balls or scouting the surroundings for certain things, themes or colors.

Pearls are from PwP

"It took me a long time to recognize it, but my diaphragm muscle was among the muscles that first lost connections. It was also discovered that I had central sleep apnea. I was informed that I was an "shallow breather" before being diagnosed with PD. It is a constant struggle to train my brain for more efficient breathing patterns." Chrystal Kafka

Just Breathe

This sounds easy enough, isn't it? However, diaphragmatic breathing is a complicated subject that is extremely valuable to patients with Parkinson's disease.

Breathing is an excellent method to remain conscious and focus while exercising or resting. Although shallow breathing may cause muscle tension, intentional and deep breathing may encourage relaxation and help make movements seem more natural. In the end, deliberate breathing is the best technique to link your brain and body.

Furthermore, breathing with a strategic approach including deep breaths as well as exhales that are long-lasting can be efficient ways to relax the nervous system, and assist to relax. The calm breath helps to prepare your brain to create positive shifts by getting the mind out the "fight or flight" mode.

Exercise Rx 1 Diaphragmatic Breathing might be wondering how to determine whether you're breathing through the diaphragm. One way to tell is to place the hands of the lower ribs of your body. Your ribs should be able to stretch out in your hands when you breathe in and to fall downwards when you exhale. Also, observe the belly expand during exhale and falls when you exhale. If you are able to breathe comfortably without straining your neck or shoulders, you're performing your breathing correctly.

Exercise Rx 2: Repetition exercise 1 but increase the exhale. Inhale, for example, for 4 counts then exhale after a count of eight. Do this 12 times before starting again if you would like to go on. This is turning into a more breathing meditation.

Exercise Rx 3: Follow through with a breathing App. Breathe2Relax has been one of my top choices. It allows you to set the duration as well as the sound and settings to receive visual signals when you breathe. It's a great way to relax.

It is evident that the diaphragm muscle is a skeletal one that forms a dome within your ribcage that is above your stomach contents.

The pelvic floor is an array of muscles which form an elongated structure that is located that is located at the bottom of your pelvis. Similar to other muscles of skeletal origin within PwP, this one might require a bit of exercise and focus to keep them fit and healthy.

If you're healthy the diaphragm as well as those muscles in the pelvic region function as an accordion. They contract each other in a fluid and flowing manner. As with any muscles in PwP, they may become disorganized weak, uncoordinated as well as tight or weak when they are not in the right places.

Pelvic floor problems can lead to pain and constipation. Regular breathing exercises that are deep and consistent with pelvic floor exercises aid in ensuring that the diaphragm as well as the pelvic floor to function and aid in reducing certain of the negative symptoms of Parkinson's.

Exercise Rx 4 diaphragmatic and breath synergization with the pelvic area If you're looking to go fancy, consider adding pelvic floor contractions into the diaphragmatic breathing exercises.

After you master your diaphragmatic breathing techniques (because you're amazing) You can then include a pelvic floor contraction on every exhale. These contractions of the pelvic floor feel similar to the sensation of a "stopping the urine flow" contraction. After that, you can relax your pelvic floor while you breathe and repeat.

If you're struggling in constipation or back pain It may be beneficial to find an PT who specializes on the pelvic floor. They're the best in the diaphragmatic and pelvic muscles' function.

Find an expert in pelvic floor rehabilitation within your region by following this page

Exercise Rx number 5: Blend breath and movement. - Think about doing exercises for your mind and body that concentrate on the integration of breath and moving. Pilates as well as yoga as well as dance are all examples of exercises for the mind which emphasize breathing in a controlled manner with movements.

The aim is to employ your breath as a method to help you move. As an example, you breathe while you increase your body, and then get larger while exhaling as you shrink your body, and shrink. Another method is to verbalize the exhale with a steady vowel sound. One way that might be easier for those suffering from Parkinson's disease, to help promote relaxation and diaphragmatic involvement is to vocalize continuous "SSSSSSSSSS" sounds with every exhale.

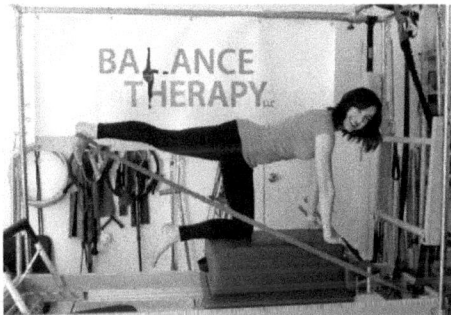

6. Exercise Rx Utilize breath to aid in switching the positions. Are you having difficulty moving from your chair? Start by taking an inhale and take a deep breath and then make a and forceful "Ssssshhhhhh!" sound and watch what transpires.

Mental Rehearsal

It's not enough to say Rehearsing and practicing movements increases body and spatial understanding within PwP. Rehearsing with your mind is an excellent technique to maintain the movement quality and improve the function of body and brain of the PwP. The only thing you need to do is set your attention on the full movements you are fond of.

Pearl of a PWP

"If you're doing a different kind of exercise, look up videos, or get someone else to show how to move to you. It is very effective to use visual cues, rather than verbal ones."

The exercise prescription: a little imagination goes far. Make sure to get as vivid as you can and truly feel the movement through your brain. Include music, if it helps. The repetition of sounds is extremely beneficial for your brain, so make sure to keep your brain active.

If I had my brain with PD I'd imagine my self doing yoga or performing dance at its highest level. Some might like to picture them playing golf. This requires the same amount of effort and commitment as any physical workout It can also provide a quick solution to improve and maintain your movement if you're at the middle of a crisis or are simply bored. If you're able to practice it enough you could find your actions and movements have significantly enhanced. You may also be able to feel a sense of calm in the mind and soul, too.

Chapter 6: What Exactly Is Parkinson's Disease?

The neurological condition Parkinson's disease is a disease that gets worse with the course of time. The substantia nerve, an area of the brain, is responsible for destroying nerve cells. Controlling the movement of a person is controlled by this part in the brain. People suffering from Parkinson's disease usually experience shaking, or abnormal motions as a result. While medications can help ease symptoms, there's no method to delay or treat the condition.

A condition of the nervous system known as Parkinson's disease impacts the area of the brain that regulates the movement. The patient may not initially notice the condition because it can develop slowly. It may start as a small shaking in your hands, nevertheless, could gradually cause an impact on your abilities to speak, walk as well as sleep.

The older you get, the more likely to suffer from the condition. It's also possible but less frequently that it could begin when you're still a teenager.

While there isn't a treatment for the disease Parkinson's you can look for treatment or assistance in order to control the signs.

How Does Parkinson's Disease Affect the Brain?

The brain's substantia-nigra region which is located in the basal ganglia found deep within. Dopamine, a neurotransmitter, that transmits signals throughout your brain is made by a subset of cells. Dopamine is a quick way to communicate to the nerve cell that regulates movement whenever you want to kick the ball or scratch an itching.

If the mechanism functions properly, your body is able to move effortlessly and in a uniform manner. Cells in your substantia-nigra begin to die when you suffer from Parkinson's disease. The levels of dopamine drop due to the inability of replenishing them that prevents your body from sending out multiple commands to regulate the smoothness of your physical movements.

Initially, you will not notice any changes. As time passes, the more your brain's functions are affected it will reach an end point, and you begin showing signs.

Parkinson's disease could occur for a long duration before you even realize because it may not be apparent until the 80 percent fibers disappear.

WHAT CAUSES THIS PROBLEM?

No one is fully aware of what causes Parkinson's disease. It is likely that a variety of factors, such as genetics or exposure to specific chemicals have contributed to the development of this disease. It's often difficult to determine the reasons why or who will purchase any item. It is rare for Parkinson's disease to run through families.

The cause for why a large number brain cells have died is still unknown to medical professionals. Though the cause isn't immediate, scientists believe that it could be the result of your genetics and the surrounding environment.

Someone who has the mutation that is linked to Parkinson's disease might never suffer from the illness. It happens frequently. Furthermore, only a small percent of those who work in places that are contaminated with substances that are linked to Parkinson's disease be diagnosed with it.

Certain neuron cells (neurons) located in the brain are gradually degraded or die due to the effects of Parkinson's disease. Loss of the neurons that make dopamine, the brain's chemical signal which is at the core of several of the signs. Dopamine deficiencies can cause an irregular brain activity that increases the risk of movement as well as other symptoms of Parkinson's disease.

The reason for Parkinson's disease remains undetermined, many elements, like the ones listed below are believed to be responsible:

* Genes. The cause of Parkinson's has been associated with certain genetic variations According to the experts. The condition is not common, however it is unlikely that a few of family members suffer from Parkinson's disease.

In contrast certain gene variants appear to raise the likelihood of having Parkinson's disease, even though the genes being associated with a lower risk of developing the disease.

• Environmental triggers of Parkinson's disease are more likely to be manifested later in life, as the result of toxic substances or environmental triggers, but the chance of developing it is low.

Chapter 7: Who Is At Risk For Parkinson's Disease?

Women and men suffer from Parkinson's disease. The disease affects men 1.5 times more frequently than females. People who are older have a higher chance of experiencing the condition. People who are younger than 50 only experience approximately 4 out of 100 cases. About 60,000 Americans discover they suffer from Parkinson's disease every year. One million people are affected in the United States and 10 million individuals worldwide are affected by this disease.

Risk Elements

The risk factors for Parkinson's disease include:

* Age. Parkinson's disease is a rare phenomenon among younger adults. The majority of cases begin in latter half of life or in the middle The risk of developing it will increase as you get older. Most people with Parkinson's disease are aged 60 and over.

Family planning decisions can help with genetic counseling in the event that someone is young and recognized as having Parkinson's. In addition to the issues of an older person with Parkinson's disease, and needing special focus are social, work situations, and the drug's negative consequences.

* Heredity. Chances of acquiring Parkinson's disease is higher if have family members in your close circle who suffer from the disease. In the absence of a substantial amount of relatives who suffer from Parkinson's disease the odds aren't that high.

* Sex. The disease is more prevalent in males often than females.

Exposure to toxic substances. Your risk of developing Parkinson's disease could increase when you're constantly exposed to herbicides or pesticides.

COMPLICATIONS

These other disorders typically present in Parkinson's disease. They are treated

1. Problems with thinking. Cognitive problems and dementia could develop in you. They are more common with Parkinson's disease, which is in advanced levels. Very rarely, do drugs help the cognitive impairments?

2. Depression and emotional stress could affect you at the beginning of its course. It is possible to handle the added issues associated with Parkinson's disease when you seek treatment for depression. It is possible that there are some other changes in your emotions including anxiety, fear or loss of motivation. The doctor may recommend medications for these signs.

3. Problems with breathing are common when the situation gets more severe. It is possible that you have difficulty swallowing. A slower swallowing pace can result in saliva accumulating in your mouth. This could cause you to drool.

4. Probleme with eating and chewing. As it progresses Parkinson's disease can affect the muscles of the mouth. This can make eating difficult. It can lead to inadequate diet and even choking.

5. Sleep disorders and trouble with Parkinson's disease sleep. Patients often are suffering from insomnia, which can manifest as regular awakenings at night in the early morning, as well as the ability to sleep during the day.

6. Quick eye motion behavioral sleep problem. This could include playing out your fantasy. The chances of sleeping better are higher if you are taking medications.

7. In Parkinson's disease, bladder problems can lead to bladder problems. This includes an inability to manage urinary frequency or difficulties in doing so.

8. Constipation. People with Parkinson's disease are often suffering from constipation due to a slower-moving digestive system.

There are other things you could meet:

* Blood pressure fluctuates as you rise suddenly, a drop in blood pressure could make people feel dizzy or lightheaded (orthostatic hypotension).

Dysfunction: can be observed. It is possible to experience issues with smell. It is possible that you have difficulty getting a scent or distinguishing different smells.

* Chronic fatigue: People with Parkinson's disease typically report feeling exhausted and drained of energy, especially at night. The reason for this may be not clear.

* Pain: A few sufferers of Parkinson's disease experience discomfort across their entire body, or in specific areas.

Sexual dysfunction Reduction in sexual desire or performance has been observed by certain Parkinson's disease sufferers.

Symptoms

The symptoms and signs of Parkinson's illness may vary between people. The early signs may be unnoticeable and even mild. If symptoms do begin with limbs that are affected on the opposite side, symptoms typically appear at one end of the body, and then become much more severe there.

A few Parkinson's symptoms and signs comprise:

* Tremor. The term "rhythmic shaking" is used for a tremor. It usually begins within a part of your body, usually within your fingers or hand. Use your thumb and fingers to rub between your thumb and fingers. The term for this is "pill-rolling tremor." The hand may tremble when in a seated position. It might stop when you're engaged in a project.

Slower motion (bradykinesia). The way you move can be affected as time passes by Parkinson's disease. This can make easy chores time-consuming and difficult. The steps you take may decrease while you move. The process of getting out of a chair can be a challenge. Your feet may shuffle and move as you walk.

* Muscles that are strong. It is possible that you have stiff muscles all over your body. The range of motion you can experience could be restricted and uncomfortable in the event that your muscles are stiff.

Poor balance and posture. Your posture may begin to slump. A condition known as Parkinson's disease can lead you to lose balance and fall.

* Automatic movements disappear. There is a possibility that you will be less able to walk if you are making unintentional motions like grinning, blinking or moving your arms.

* Speech changes. The option is talking softly, quickly speaking in a slur, pausing, or tumbling. The typical patterns of speech used by you may not be included in your voice, which might be monotonous.

Writing improves. The writing process can become difficult Your writing may seem small.

Things to be aware of

Parkinson's disease is progressively worse. Also it is likely that your symptoms get worse over time. Individually your Parkinson's symptoms may differ in a significant way. They may also differ regarding how fast it progresses and how severe it gets. It is possible to ignore or deny the first symptoms. The symptoms may start with one side of your body and then switch over to the opposite side.

Chapter 8: What Is The Specific Of What My Doctor Will Look At?

In the case of Parkinson's disease, there isn't one test for Parkinson's disease. Most of the time, it is based on your signs and the medical history, but it can take some time to establish. This method involves excluding any other diseases that can are similar to Parkinson's disease. A doctor may perform an MRI dating scan in order to search for dopamine levels in the brain. It may help in diagnosing.

Because there isn't a single testing method, it is crucial that you speak to an expert in the subject matter as fast as is possible. It's simple to miss.

If you're also affected then your physician may employ this Hoehn or Yahr scale to evaluate the level of disease you're in. The scale evaluates the degree of the symptoms you are experiencing between 1 and 5, where 5 is the severest.

Knowing the stages will aid in determining what you can be expecting as the disease progresses and also where the symptoms of yours can be categorized. But, keep in mind that certain people may experience mild to severe symptoms in the course of 20 to 30 years. Other people go through changes quicker.

Prevention

The cause of Parkinson's disease is not clear There aren't any proven ways to stop it.

Regular aerobic exercise can help decrease the risk of having Parkinson's disease according to numerous studies.

Based on other studies that found those who drink caffeine, which is found in drinks like tea, coffee as well as soda, were at an lower chance of getting Parkinson's disease. The risk of developing Parkinson's disease has been linked to the consumption of green tea. Caffeine could be linked to Parkinson's disease in a different manner, but this remains a matter of the debate. It is currently not enough evidence to back up the assertion that consumption of drinks with caffeine may aid in preventing the development of Parkinson's illness.

Is Surgery a Possibility?

Deep brain stimulation could be recommended by your doctor in the event that your medication is not working (DBS). Doctors must place electrodes in the brain to induce DBS. An attached device transmits electrical signals to them. These electrical pulses can be beneficial for controlling the tremors of Parkinson's.

In the past, doctors employed various procedures to harm the brain in order in order to treat disorders of movement. The procedures have been used infrequently today.

What will this illness do to me personally?

Parkinson's disease can change an individual's life but the majority of people live regular or nearly normal lives.

In some cases, medication helps to reduce symptoms and they're usually not severe. Certain illnesses of patients are more serious and severely limit their ability to perform.

The daily routines of taking a bath and driving to work can be difficult when it gets more difficult. Writing can be difficult assignment. The later stages can lead to dementia.

While Parkinson's disease could have a profound impact on your daily lifestyle, you are able to take part in the activities you love when you have the appropriate treatment and assistance by your medical team. It's crucial to seek out relatives and friends to help. Making sure that you receive support is an essential to living with Parkinson's disease.

PARKINSON'S DISEASE AND DIET

Levodopa (Sinemet) and bromocriptine (Parlodel) are frequently employed to treat symptoms of Parkinson's disease. Yet, there is no way to remove the symptoms.

There are some who may consider alternative therapies as there isn't a treatment for the disease, and medications used to treat the symptoms could have adverse effects.

Although certain diet changes can aid some individuals suffering from symptoms of Parkinson's disease nutritional changes alone are not able to cure the illness.

The experts are looking into methods to boost dopamine levels by consuming a balanced diet, since the condition is linked to a lack of dopamine cell types in the body.

Additionally, changes in lifestyle such as exercising and eating healthier can aid in the treatment of other symptoms associated with Parkinson's disease, such as dementia and confusion.

Foods that are rich in antioxidants can also help reduce the oxidative stress that occurs in the brain. This can cause some degeneration of the brain that occurs in patients with Parkinson's disease.

Fiber supplements and probiotics can help with constipation as well Another possible symptom however, the evidence for this is mixed.

Additionally, in spite of the dearth evidence to support it, supplementing magnesium could help alleviate Parkinson's disease-related muscular cramps. But, insufficient levels of magnesium are believed as a factor that contributes to the onset of Parkinson's disease. Therefore, the importance of magnesium.

Foods that can help with the treatment of Parkinson's disease

While the research is unfinished and unclear some studies have focused on flavonoids, proteins, as well as gut flora in order to decrease the symptoms of Parkinson's disease.

Further research has proven that diets with antioxidants can benefit the brain as well as slow the progress of Alzheimer's disease among older adults.

Antioxidants

Antioxidants help prevent the oxidative stress that is a common occurrence during Parkinson's illness as a consequence of a mismatch between antioxidants and free radicals.

They are brimming with antioxidants.

Nuts can include walnuts Brazil nuts, pecans and pistachios.

The berries include things such as blackberries, blueberries, the goji berries and cranberries and elderberries.

The vegetables of the night include peppers, eggplants and tomatoes.

The most common leafy greens include spinach and kale.

The most antioxidant-rich diet could result from a plant-based diet rich in these food groups.

The treatment of antioxidants is a different subject of research for those suffering from Parkinson's disease. However, the results are only preliminary.

Flava beans

Due to the fact that fava beans have levodopa, which is a chemical found in many Parkinson's medicines Many people take them for treating the disease. It's not clear of how these beans can help treat the symptoms of Parkinson's disease, but.

Fava beans should not be utilized to replace prescription medicines since you cannot determine what amount of levodopa is coming from them.

food items high in omega-3

In patients with Parkinson's disease the omega-3 fatty acids, an unhealthy fat, could help boost brain performance. Some foods may contain the fats.

* salmon\halibut\oysters

* Soy beans are made from soy

* beans containing flaxseed, and kidneys

According to research studies according to some research, according to some studies, the Mediterranean diet, packed with omega-3 fatty acids, antioxidants and other could help those suffering from Parkinson's disease to prevent the development of dementia.

Several nutrient-dense foods

Cognitive impairment is connected to malnutrition as an danger aspect. Additionally, malnutrition is most likely to be present when people suffer from Parkinson's disease.

This list of foods that are suitable for those suffering from Parkinson's disease are deficient in the following essential nutrients:

Tofu, beef, spinach and breakfast cereals fortified with iron include examples of foods that are rich in iron.

Vitamin B1 is found in abundance in pork, beans peas and lentils.

Red meat, whole grains oysters, chicken, and red meat are among the foods rich in zinc.

Tuna, salmon and fortified dairy items as well as the cod liver oil a few sources of food products that are rich in vitamin D.

Dairy items and leafy vegetables as well as fortified soybean products are the best sources of calcium.

The things to be wary of If you suffer from Parkinson's disease

It is possible to restrict your consumption of certain food items in the event that you suffer from Parkinson's disease.

Foods that are saturated with fatty acids

While the exact role played by saturated fats in the development of Parkinson's disease remains unclear but research indicates that consuming large amounts of fat in your food can increase the risk of contracting the disease.

High-fat diets are often linked with health issues like heart disease and chronic inflammation. There is a possibility that you should eat them in moderate quantities in order to avoid.

The foods that are high in saturated fat comprise:

certain baked and fried food items butter, cow lard, dairy products, palm oil and cheese

There is a small amount of evidence indicates that some Parkinson's sufferers could benefit from a fat-rich ketogenic diet. However the low-fat diet can have advantages. It is generally true that more study is required.

Chapter 9: Tips For Living Well With Parkinson's

Here are a few simple adjustments to lifestyles that can help lessen the signs of Parkinson's disease

Take a large amount of water. Patients with Parkinson's should drink a lot of water as they may not show the typical signs of thirst. Consume 6 to 8 complete glass (1.2 to 1.6 milliliters) of water every day for optimal health.

Get outside and take some time. Inhaling some sunlight and fresh air can reduce the symptoms of Parkinson's disease, as vitamin D's been found to help fight the disease.

Make sure you are moving your feet. You may improve your abilities by certain kinds of physical therapy could reduce the development of Parkinson's disease.

Consider taking vitamins. Talk to your physician about possibilities of supplements or other therapies that might be suitable for you.

6 WAYS TO FEEL BETTER WITHOUT MEDICATION IF YOU HAVE PARKINSON'S

In the case of people suffering from Parkinson's disease, there are many strategies they can employ alongside medication to improve the health of their bodies and improve their physical performance, decrease symptoms and improve their overall quality of life. A regular exercise routine, healthy diet, drinking plenty of fluids and getting enough rest are among the most important.

However, what are the alternatives to traditional therapies? The interest in treating Parkinson's disease has increased with time due to the advent of holistic therapies like massage, yoga, diet supplements, as well as other types of therapy for movement. A variety of non-medical therapies are promising however, the jury remains to be decided on a few of these.

Take a look at the following treatment options:

Supplements for Nutrition

You're probably aware of anyone that antioxidant coenzyme Q10commonly called Co-Q10, can assist in the treatment of Parkinson's disease. In 2011 in 2011, the National Institute of Neurological Disorders and Stroke took the decision to stop studying the effectiveness of coenzymeQ10 once it was discovered that the claimed preventative advantages of coenzyme Q10 weren't distinct from the benefits of the placebo.

It is vital to talk with your doctor prior to the use of a supplement to treat this and many other reasons. Additionally, you must always adhere to your prescription medicine.

Since many of the foods packed with calcium (such as dairy products) contain proteins, and this can interfere in absorption of drug taking calcium supplements could be beneficial for people suffering from Parkinson's disease.

Tai Chi

There is a reason to believe that patients with Parkinson's disease would be able to benefit from this type of activity since it enhances balance as well as coordination. Tai Chi, resistance exercise as well as stretching have been proven to improve balance and stability for those suffering from moderate Parkinson's disease. The study found that Tai Chi was the most effective among these three types of exercises.

The patients with Parkinson's have a significant impairment in balance. This leads to the loss of their capacity to perform tasks as well as an increased chance of falling. It is frequently suggested by doctors However, only a few routines have proven to be effective.

Patients suffering from Parkinson's disease idiopathic participated in a random and controlled test to find out whether an tai chi program specially designed to help them aid in improving their postural stability. A total of

195 people suffering from Hoehn and Yahr stages 1 through 4 of the disease were randomly placed into one of three classes: Tai chi and weight-training, as well as stretching. Patients participated in workout sessions of 60 minutes every week, for a period of 24 weeks. The variations in the limitations-of-stability test from initial results were used as a key indicator of their success (maximum excitation and the control of direction; between 0 and 100 percent). The rate of falls as well as evaluations of gait and strength were additionally assessed as secondary outcomes as well as the results of functional reach, test of timed up-and go as well as motor scores from the Unified Parkinson's Disease Rating Scale and functional reaching.

Yoga

It has been proven that yoga can improve balance and flexibility, as well as those with Parkinson's disease might see the same benefits. An investigation conducted in 2012 found that yoga can improve the strength, balance, mobility as well as flexibility, especially in the case of a practice that is specifically designed to meet those suffering from mobility disorders, such as Parkinson's disease. Yoga can also boost the quality of your sleep and mood.

Massage Treatment

Although the advantages of massage therapy in decreasing the negative consequences of Parkinson's disease prominent tremors are apparent but the treatment isn't durable. A study conducted in 2016 of the research found that a 60 minute massage reduced tension in muscles as well as resting shaking.

Chapter 10: Therapy Based On Movement

Parkinson's disease that affects balance and leads to a gradual loss of motor skills could have some symptoms eased by the help of certain movements therapy. Patients with Parkinson's disease who use Alexander Technique Alexander Technique, for instance might find it simpler to maintain their mobility.

A different approach that seeks to help the body learn to be able to do the difficult movements includes one of the methods known as Feldenkrais Method. Even if you do not take part at "official" movement therapies, workouts like dancing and strengthening exercises (using machines or weights) could help alleviate some signs. Check with your doctor prior to beginning an exercise program.

Acupuncture

The basic idea behind Chinese medical practices that rely on Acupuncture is that it simulates the meridians throughout the body (or energy pathways) can provide benefits, including the relief of pain. This is why the practice is widely utilized to treat Parkinson's diseases in China as well as other countries.

People who regularly take it throughout the United States say it helps in reducing fatigue and sleep disturbances. Even though acupuncture can be considered neuroprotective during research on animals (slowing the loss of neuronal cells that cause Parkinson's disease) However, the outcomes haven't been proven for humans.

The treatments could also prove beneficial.

It is possible to learn how exercises are performed that are part of physical therapy to increase the strength and stability of your body and help maintain your self-sufficiency. Learn new methods for doing your daily chores through occupational therapy. Speech therapy can be beneficial in cases of choppy or slow speech.

Exercise and nutrition

Foods that are nutritious can lift your spirits. It can also assist with symptoms of Parkinson's disease, such as constipation. In addition, regular exercise can improve your flexibility, balance and endurance. Request your physician to suggest the services of a physical therapist, or an workout regimen.

The key is managing symptoms. The muscles that are tight, tremors and slow movements can be treated with Parkinson's medications. The doctor may also recommend occupational therapy, physical therapy or speech therapy based the way you respond. Surgery may be required in some instances.

Dopamine-producing drugs are employed in treatment.

Parkinson's disease can affect the dopamine-producing nerve cells in the brain. Therefore, the chemical levels drop. Levodopa is commonly employed by physicians to initiate the treatment (L-dopa). Your brain changes it into dopamine. In order to manage the side negative effects, you'll probably use it in conjunction with another medication known as carbidopa, since it can cause you to feel sick on your stomach. This drug-drug combination is often known as carbidopa-levodopa (Parcopa, Rytary, Sinemet).

Treatment: Increasing the Effects of Dopamine

Any of these in its own or when used in conjunction with another medication, could be prescribed by your doctor:

Dopamine antagonists: They provide similar effects to dopamine, but they do not increase the concentration of dopamine in the brain. Levodopa-containing drugs can be used in conjunction together. Consider pramipexole or ropinirole (Mirapex) (Requip).

COMT Inhibitors: They increase the effect of levodopa. Entacapone (Comtan) or tolcapone can be prescribed directly to the user (Tasmar).

Levodopa does not break into your brain via MAO-B inhibitors. Rasagiline and selegiline

(Eldepryl, Zelapar) are two alternatives (Azilect).

These drugs are prescribed for treating tremors.

In order to treat Parkinson's disease-related movements The doctor might also suggest treatment. These drugs, often known as anticholinergics are used to block the brain's neurotransmitter which regulates the movement. Trihexyphenidyl, or benztropine mesylate (Cogentin) can be used (Artane).

WHICH FOODS TO EAT IF YOU HAVE PARKINSON'S DISEASE

An energizing diet can improve overall health, and improves you manage illness signs. In order to stay active and fit, it is essential to drink plenty of water and consume various meals that are complete like vegetables, fruits Lean protein, whole grains, beans and legumes.

Parkinson's sufferers must make an enormous amount of work to keep their fitness and strength. Based on research, changing your life style can assist you to attain two goals:

Improved control of symptom.

* The disease progresses slowly.

The focus on fitness and food choices can be:

* Maintain good overall health over the long term.

Help you avoid complications of Parkinson's disease, such as constipation.

Increase your mobility and balance.

Improve the level of your existence.

Chapter 11: Parkinson's Disease

It is known as a brain-related degenerative disease that causes your brain to become degraded when you age. Errors and slow movement imbalance issues, as well as others are typical. A majority of cases occur due to unknown reasons however, some cases are inherited. While the condition isn't treatable, there are many alternatives to treat it.

What causes Parkinson's disease?

Parkinson's disease can be described as a condition that causes a part of the brain becomes degraded as time passes, resulting in more severe signs. Although this disease is most commonly identified for its impact on the control of muscles as well as balance and movement but it also impacts the ability to think, your senses as well as your mental health and various other areas of your everyday life.

Who's affected?

Parkinson's disease is more likely become more prevalent as you age and the average start-up age of sixty years old. Males or those who are designated to be males at birth (DMAB) have a slight higher susceptible than women and those who are designated as female at birth (WDMAB) (DFAB).

Although Parkinson's disease is usually linked to old age but it may affect adults younger than 20. (though this is extremely uncommon as a lot of people have a sibling, parent or parent who suffers from the same disease).

How prevalent is this ailment?

Parkinson's disease is one of the most prevalent age-related degenerative brain disease, which ranks 2nd. This is also the most prevalent motor-related brain disease that affects. Researchers estimate that around one percent of those who are over 60 suffer from the disorder worldwide.

What impact does this condition affect my body?

The basal ganglia (a brain part) of the brain to shrink. The brain loses the capabilities that you had previously in this part of the brain because it is deteriorating. The disease of Parkinson causes a dramatic shift in brain chemical, as per research.

The neurotransmitters in the brain utilizes to regulate how neurons (neurons) communicate to one another under regular situations. Parkinson's disease can be caused by the absence of dopamine, one of the vital neurotransmitters.

The brain transmits activated signals to muscles for movement, the cells requiring dopamine adjust the actions you perform. The symptoms of Parkinson's disease include slow motions and tremors. These result from a deficiency of dopamine.

The signs and symptoms of Parkinson's disease get worse when the disease progresses. Depression and symptoms resembling dementia are typical in the latter stages of the disease which affect the way your brain performs.

What is the distinction between Parkinson's disease and Parkinson's?

The term "pilgrim" is used to describe a broad range of symptoms for the disease Parkinson's and any others with similar signs. It is a term that can refer to many different conditions, like multiple system atrophy as well as corticobasal degeneration in addition to Parkinson's disease.

What are the warning signs and indications?

Control issues with muscles are one of the Parkinson's disease's most widely-known signs. The experts now understand that difficulties in muscle control aren't necessarily the only signs of Parkinson's disease.

Movement-related symptoms

The motor manifestations of Parkinson's disease, also known as movement-related symptoms, consist of the following symptoms:

* Movements that are slower (bradykinesia). This sign is necessary for the diagnosis of Parkinson's disease. The people suffering from this disease describe the condition as weakness of muscles, but it's caused by muscles control issues, not weakness.

* A tremor which occurs in muscles that are at still. The tremor is an erratic shake of the muscles even when they're not being employed, and is seen in about 80percent of Parkinson's disease instances. Essential tremors rarely happen when muscles are their rest. However, the resting tremors can occur.

* Resilience or stiffness. Parkinson's disease manifests itself as Cogwheel stiffness and lead-pipe rigidity. If a part of the body is moved that has lead-pipe rigidity, it remains constant and unchanging stiffness. When lead-pipe stiffness and tremor is combined, stiffness of the cogwheel is created. The fast, stop-and-go nature of these movements is

what creates its nickname (think that it is the second-hand on the mechanical clock).

A gait or posture that is unstable in walking. The disease of Parkinson causes a posture that is slouched or stooped due to slow movements and stiffness. The signs typically show up with the progression of the condition. When someone walks, you can see that they walk with shorter, shuffle movements and are using the arms more. The steps may be long in a walk.

Other possible motor signposts include:

* I'm blinking more than I would normally. It's also an indication that facial muscles are not as strong.

* Handwriting that is cramped, or small. The condition is that is caused by the muscle imbalance.

* Drooling. Another indication that is seen as facial muscle control becomes reduced.

* Face that has a mask-like expression. The expressions of faces vary very barely or none anyhow, and this is called hypomimia.

It is difficult to swallow (dysphagia). A decreased control of the throat muscles can cause this. This increases the chance of issues like pneumonia and the risk of choking.

A voice that's very soft (hypophonia). It is the result from a decrease in muscle control within the chest and neck.

Chapter 12: Non-Movement Symptoms

Additionally, there are symptoms that don't have anything to do with the movement of muscles or their control. These symptoms weren't previously thought to as risk factors for this condition when they first appeared prior to the symptoms of motor. There is now increasing evidence to suggest that these signs could be present early in process of progression. This means that these signs could signal early warning signs that manifest several years, even decades before the first motor-related symptoms occur.

There are a few non-motor signs (with the possibility of early warning signs):

* Signs and symptoms of the autonomic nervous systems Orthostatic hypotension (low blood pressure while standing) constipation, digestive problems, urinary incontinence and sexual problems are but some of the symptoms.

* Depression.

* Sensory loss (anosmia).

* Periodic motion disorder (PLMD) Rapid eye movement (REM) behavioral disorder as well as restless legs syndrome, are all sleep disorders.

* The disease of Parkinson's can cause difficulty in focusing and thinking.

Parkinson's Disease Stages

The disease of Parkinson could take a long time in some cases, even decades for it to develop. Margaret Hoehn and Melvin Yahr Two experts created the Parkinson's disease staging method in the year 1967. Because staging for this condition isn't as beneficial as knowing the way it affects each individual's lives individually and treating them in a way that is appropriate, the system has ceased to be extensively employed.

The Movement Disorder Society's Unified Parkinson's Disease Rating Scale (MDS-UPDRS) is currently the main method used by health professionals to diagnose Parkinson's disease. The MDS-UPDRS examines four distinct aspects of Parkinson's disease.

Part 1: Non-motor components of daily life. Non-motor (non-movement) indicators such as depression, dementia, anxiety and various mental capacity as well as mental health issues are covered in this segment. The section also addresses discomfort, constipation, urinary exhaustedness, incontinence, as well as other problems.

Part 2: Motor aspects that are part of our daily lives. Effects of movements on activities and skills are addressed in this chapter. If you have tremors they affect your ability to talk, eat chew, swallow and so on in addition to the capacity to wash and dress oneself.

Motor examination is the final element. It is utilized by health professionals to assess the impact of movement on Parkinson's disease. The test criteria consider the way you speak and your facial expressions rigidity and stiffness, your speed and walking patterns and balance, motion speed, as well as the tremors you experience, in addition to other factors.

Fourth Part: Motor issues An expert will evaluate the extent to which the signs of Parkinson's disease have an impact on the way you live your life. This will include both the amount of you are suffering from specific signs and symptoms every day, as well as how they impact the way you use your time.

What is the cause of this disease?

In spite of the fact that there are a variety of recognized risk factors that can cause Parkinson's disease, including exposure to pesticides, the sole confirmed cause of Parkinson's disease is genetic. If Parkinson's disease doesn't occur due to a genetic change is referred to as "idiopathic" (which means "on its own" in Greek). It means they don't have any clue as to why the disease occurs.

There are many symptoms that resemble those of Parkinson's disease, but they are in fact parkinsonism (a expression used for

Parkinson's similar symptoms) result from a particular factor, for instance the use of certain medications for psychiatric disorders.

Family members with Parkinson's disease

The disease of Parkinson can be passed down through families. That means you may be affected by the parents or one of them. But, it only accounts about 10% of the cases.

A minimum of seven genes have been identified as being linked to Parkinson's disease, according to researchers. Three are linked to the disease's onset early (meaning the disease is more advanced than normal age). Genetic mutations can result in specific features.

Parkinson's disease is caused by an unknown source

Idiopathic Parkinson's disease, as per to medical experts, is caused due to issues with the way the body process the protein - synuclein (alpha si-nu-clein). Proteins are chemical molecules that have an distinctive form. The misfolding of proteins happens when certain proteins aren't in the proper structure and aren't able to be used or broken down by the body.

The accumulation of proteins occurs in a variety of areas or within certain cells due to the fact that they do not have a place to move (tangles or in clumps made in these protein clumps are known as Lewy body). The growth of Lewy bodies causes toxic results and even cell death (which is not associated as a result of some genetic disorders that lead to the disease Parkinson's).

The misfolding of proteins is known to be a factor in many different illnesses, such as Huntington's Disease, Alzheimer's as well as various forms of amyloidosis.

The condition has been linked to Parkinsonism.

Some experts have linked specific instances or situations with parkinsonism. Even though these disorders aren't necessarily Parkinson's disease, they have some of the same signs, and doctors might consider them in diagnosing the disease.

Here are a few potential causes:

* Medications. Many drugs mimic effects of Parkinson's disease. If you stop using the medication that causes the effects of Parkinson's disease prior to them becoming permanent, symptoms generally disappear. But, the effects of the medication can persist for several weeks or months following the time you stopped using it.

* Encephalitis. The condition, also known as brain inflammation may cause parkinsonism in certain people.

* Toxins and poisons. Parkinsonism may be triggered through a myriad of causes like manganese dust carbon monoxide and welding gases and insects.

Injury has caused harm. The brain injury may be the result of frequent head injuries like those that occur during intense contact sports such as football, boxing or hockey. It is referred to as "post-traumatic parkinsonism."

Are they infected?

Parkinson's disease isn't communicable and is not a disease that can be transmitted from another person.

What does it mean to be identified?

It is typically diagnosed with a medical procedure where a medical professional assesses your symptoms, questions your questions and goes over the medical history of you. Certain diagnostic tests and lab tests are offered, but they're usually used to determine if you have other diseases or cause. The majority of blood tests don't need to be taken except if you're not responding to treatments for Parkinson's disease this could mean you've an additional illness.

What kinds of tests can be conducted to determine the severity the condition?

Different diagnostic and imaging tests are accessible to health professionals who suspect the presence of Parkinson's disease, or who want to determine if there are other conditions. They include:

* Blood tests (these will help to rule out any other types of parkinsonism).

* CT scan (computerized tomography).

* Genetic analysis

* Imaging using magnet resonance (MRI).

* PET scan (positron emission tomography).

It is possible to create innovative laboratory tests.

Researchers have come up with viable methods to detect Parkinson's disease signs. These two tests are based on the alpha-synuclein proteins and are different in their approaches. Although these tests can't identify the conditions are the result of improperly folded alpha-synuclein proteins however, they will aid your physician in determining an appropriate diagnosis.

The procedures used during both tests follow the following steps.

• Tap your spinal cord. One of these tests checks at the presence of alpha-synuclein proteins that are misfolded the cerebrospinal fluid surrounding the spinal cord and brain. The spinal tap (lumbar puncture) is a method that involves a doctor who places a needle inside your spinal canal to gather cerebrospinal fluid to test.

The skin is a good place to biopsy. A skin biopsy that examines the surface nerve tissue could be another test. The procedure that requires taking a little portion of your skin which includes nerves. An area on your back as well as two places in your leg were utilized for the collection of sample. The samples will then be examined to determine if the alpha-synuclein in your body contains a problem that may increase your chance of developing Parkinson's disease.

Chapter 13: How Is It Treated?

At present we have a number of choices to treat symptoms. The treatment options can differ between individuals depending on the individual ailments and the effectiveness of specific treatments. The most commonly used treatment for this condition is medicine.

The procedure of implanting devices that deliver a small amount of electrical energy to an area of the brain can be a second treatment alternative (this is referred to as deep brain stimulation). There are several experimental options for stem cells-based treatment, but the availability differs widely and a majority of them are not accessible to people with Parkinson's disease.

What medications or treatments are currently being utilized?

There are two kinds of treatment for Parkinson's disease. Direct treatment and symptomatic treatment. The disease can be treated in a direct manner. The treatment for symptoms is merely focused on the symptoms of Parkinson's disease.

Medications

Parkinson's disease medicines are effective in many methods. In the end, medicines which perform any one of the following tasks will most likely to:

* Dopamine supplementation. Levodopa and other medications can enhance the quantity of dopamine that your brain produces. If the drug isn't working typically, it's a sign that you have another type of parkinsonism and not Parkinson's disease. Levodopa long-term use can cause negative side effects which reduce its efficacy.

* Dopamine emulation. Dopamine agonists are substances that replicate the effect of dopamine. When a dopamine molecule binds on a cell, it prompts it to behave to a certain manner. Dopamine agonists may bind to cells, causing they to respond in a similar way.

Levodopa's onset delay is more common among the younger age group.

Blockers of the metabolism of dopamine. The natural processes that occur in your body reduce neurotransmitters, such as dopamine. Drugs that block the body from breaking down dopamine allows the brain to release more dopamine. They can be very beneficial early but they also assist in the later phases of Parkinson's disease when coupled with levodopa.

* Blockers of the levodopa metabolism. These medicines help your body process levodopa less quickly which allows it to last longer. As these medicines can trigger negative side effects that can harm the liver, they must be handled with care. They are frequently utilized to complement levodopa, as it becomes less efficient.

* Adenosine blockers. If used in conjunction with levodopa medication that inhibits how cells make use of Adenosine (a chemical that

is found in a variety of types all over the body) could be beneficial.

A variety of medications are offered to treat people with Parkinson's disease. The following signs are often managed:

Erectile and sexual problems.

* Fatigue or sleepiness.

* Constipation.

* Sleep problems.

* Depression.

* Dementia.

* Anxiety.

Additional psychotic signs may include hallucinations.

The stimulation of the brain at a deeper and deep

Surgery was once an option to deliberately damage and causing scarring to a part of the brain affected by Parkinson's disease. Deep brain stimulation, which uses implants to deliver an electrically moderate current in the same areas and achieves similar results.

Deep brain stimulation offers the significant benefit of being reversible while intentional damage to the brain can't be. This treatment is nearly always accessible in the latter stages of Parkinson's disease after which levodopa therapy has become no more effective, or in those who have tremors that do not appear to be a reaction to the standard medications.

Experimental treatments

The possibility of other treatment options for Parkinson's disease are currently being researched by research scientists. Although they aren't widely available but they offer the possibility of a cure for people suffering with this disease. Here are a few techniques for experimental treatment:

*Transplantation of stem cells. They replace the damaged neurons that use dopamine within your brain with brand new ones.

Treatments for healing neuron. These therapies aim to heal damaged neurons, while encouraging the development of new ones.

* Treatments and therapies targeted at genes. Particular mutations responsible for Parkinson's diseases are treated with these medications. They also aid in ensuring that levodopa and other drugs work better.

The possibility of a side effect that is that may be a result of treatment

Side effects and complications with the treatment for Parkinson's disease vary according to the treatment and the degree of illness, related health problems that you suffer from, and many other variables. Your physician is the ideal source of information about possible adverse results and the effects. They will also be able to advise you about ways to minimize the effects of such adverse effects in your daily living.

Additional information about levodopa

Levodopa is the most well-known and effective Parkinson's disease treatment. Due to the way it functions it has significantly enhanced the treatment for Parkinson's disease. However, it is recommended that doctors are cautious when using it. The majority of them prescribe various drugs to boost the efficacy of levodopa, or to ease the symptoms and side effects.

Levodopa is often mixed with other medicines to stop the drug from processing by the body prior to it can reach the brain. This can help you stay clear of other negative effects of dopamine, such as nausea, vomiting and the low blood pressure you experience in the event of standing (orthostatic hypotension).

How your body utilizes levodopa changes over time and its effectiveness may decrease. The increase in dosage can help but also raises the risk and severity of negative effects. Moreover, dosage is only able to be increased as that it is no longer safe.

What can I do to take care of myself, or manage manifestations?

It's not something it is possible to determine it isn't something you can do to manage the symptoms of Parkinson's disease without consulting with a physician.

What speed will I be feeling more energized after treatment? Also, what time will it take for to get back?

The amount of time is required to recuperate and see the effects of treatment for Parkinson's disease depends on the treatment method and the degree of illness, as well as other aspects. Additional information about what you can get from the treatment process can be gotten from your health care physician. Their information may take into consideration the unique features that could affect your treatment.

What should I do to decrease my risk of getting the risk of developing this disease?

Parkinson's disease can be caused by unpredictability or genetic causes. The disease cannot be prevented and neither can the chance of developing it be decreased. The welding and the farming industries are two jobs that carry a lot of risk, but it is not the case that everyone working in these areas is prone to developing parkinsonism.

What should I expect when I'm diagnosed with the disease?

It is known as a chronic disease meaning that its impact on the brain get worse as time passes. But, it can take some time before the condition begins to become more severe. This is why the majority of individuals live their lives as normal.

It's likely that you'll need little or little assistance initially and can be able to live on your own. When symptoms get worse and you require medication for managing the discomfort. Many drugs, especially levodopa, can be extremely or moderately effective after your doctor has determined the most effective dose for your condition.

Most of the effects and symptoms can be treated, however, as time goes by, treatments become ineffective and become more challenging. With the progress of the illness it becomes ever more challenging.

Chapter 14: What's The Outlook Of Parkinson's Disease?

While Parkinson's disease isn't fatal, its signs and consequences are often deadly. In the year 1967, an average life expectancy of people with Parkinson's disease was under 10 years. Since then, average lifespan has risen approximately 55% and now stands at nearly 14.5 years. That, in conjunction with the nature of Parkinson's disease being much more prevalent after the age of 60suggests that it is rare for the disease to shorten the duration of your life less than a couple of years (depending upon the expected life span in your area).

What should I do to take care of my self?

If you're suffering from Parkinson's disease, the best option is to follow the advice of your physician on self-care.

• Take your medication in the manner prescribed. The use of your medication as directed will significantly lessen the signs that Parkinson's diseases cause. Follow the directions for your medication and inform your physician when you suffer from any side reactions or notice that your medications aren't functioning effectively.

* If prescribed, visit your doctor. Your doctor will arrange appointments for you. These appointments are essential for helping you manage symptoms as well as determining appropriate dosages and medications.

The signs and symptoms should not be dismissed or omitted. The disease of Parkinson can trigger a range of symptoms, many of which are manageable by treating the disease, or the signs. Treatment may make a big improvement in stopping symptoms from being worsened.

Who can be affected by Parkinson's condition?

Most cases of Parkinson's are not known to medical professionals. About 10% of cases are genetically inherited, which means it is passed down through either or more parents. The rest of them therefore are considered idiopathic. This is to say they happen for unidentified motives.

What are the Parkinson's disease's early indicators of warning?

Motor (movement-related) signs like the sluggishness of movements, tremors or stiffness could be indicators of Parkinson's condition. These symptoms can, however, appear as non-motor signs. There are many non-motor signs that can develop in the years, or even years, prior to the onset of motor symptoms show. The non-motor signs, on the contrary, are unclear, making it challenging to determine if they are related to Parkinson's illness.

These non-motor signs might be indicators of early warning:

The autonomic nervous system include constipation as well as feeling lightheaded when standing up (orthostatic hypotension).

* Loss of smell sense (anosmia).

* PLMD, also known as periodic limb movement disorder (PLMD) and rapid eye movement (REM) behavioral disorder as well as restless legs syndrome, are all sleep disorders.

Are Parkinson's diseases fatal?

Parkinson's disease is not fatal by itself. However, it can be a contributing factor to other, potential fatal ailments or issues.

Home Treatments for Parkinson's Symptoms

Parkinson's disease is a condition that can make everyday living difficult. However, there are simple solutions at home that will help reduce the effects of the condition.

The disease of Parkinson's causes stiffness in the muscles as well as tremors, weakness and muscle stiffness and tremors, making daily routines difficult, particularly when the disorder progresses. Dyskinesia is one of the side effects of Parkinson's medications that results in the movement to become distorted and difficult to control. Making bathing, dressing and even walking around at residence can cause frustration.

According to the Michael J. Fox Foundation for Parkinson's Research exercising is an essential element in reducing the diseases symptoms. If you suffer from Parkinson's disease swimming or dancing, yoga and walking are all great ways to ensure that your muscles remain flexible.

"Exercise is being studied as a potential intervention and neuro [brain] protective strategy," states Linda Pituch, patient services director for the Parkinson's Disease Foundation. "It's not conclusive, but exercise could end up being considered in the same way that medication is viewed - as a treatment that you don't skip."

Stiff Muscle Stretching for Parkinson's Disease

Stretching and flexibility exercises provided below will help loosen stiff muscles, improve flexibility, and make day-to-day work easier

1. Sit about 8 inches from the wall and extend your arms upwards. For stability, rest your hands against the wall. Then, extend your arms back and up.

2. Set your back on a wall as a support, and then move at a rapid pace by raising your knees the highest is possible.

3. Spread your arms out to the side in a seat using a straight, high back. Push your shoulders forward as much as you are able to. Lift your head towards the ceiling as you extend.

4. Step your feet forward and down while you pump your arms up and down in your thighs while sitting in the chair.

To Make Medicines Work Better, Eat Less Protein

Food choices can affect the way your medication manages common Parkinson's symptoms, including shaking (uncontrollable shaking) as well as constipation.

For instance, a diet that is rich in protein may hinder your body's ability absorb levodopa, a component of Sinemet the most common Parkinson's disease medication. This is why some physicians advise patients suffering from Parkinson's disease not to consume more than 12 percent the calories they consume daily in protein. As per the Parkinson's Disease Foundation, taking the medication on empty stomach prior to meals helps in the absorption of the medication.

Not eating certain foods like:

1. Fish and meats which have been dried, cured fermented or dried

2. Seasoned cheese (cheddar blue cheese Camembert)

3. The fermentation of cabbage (sauerkraut or Kimchi)

4. Soy-based items (tofu Soy sauce, tofu)

5. Red wine and beer

6. Iron supplements (separate the iron supplements from your dosage by 2 hours or greater)

Additionally the inclusion of fruits and veggies within your diet can help to protect nerve cell activity as well as manage Parkinson's symptoms. Fruits and vegetables that contain fiber will help stimulate intestinal movement, and also reduce constipation. In order to make it easier for you to adhere to a healthy diet, talk to your doctor for recommendations to the nutritionist.

Balance Training Through Gait

Patients suffering from Parkinson's disease could benefit from home "gait training." It involves experimenting with various methods of standing, walking or change. Training participants in gait should be able to

1. While walking straight ahead make sure you take big steps and have good heel-toe alignment.

2. If you are walking or turning around when walking, ensure that your legs are about 10 inches apart for additional support. This will reduce the risk of falling.

3. The soles of shoes with rubber soles must be avoided as they could stick to the floor and create a higher risk of being thrown off.

4. Be sure to keep a steady pace when walking.

Utilizing a metronome that musicians employ to maintain the beat, it is a good way to exercise gait. An article released in PLoS One in March 2010 observed that walking to beat of a metronome approximately 10% faster than their speediest stride drastically enhanced gait of patients suffering from Parkinson's disease.

Staying safe at home with Parkinson's

Making small changes in your surroundings will help you function better when trying to manage Parkinson's disease. Health care providers, as per Pituch they can aid you with establishing a specific program to live safely as well as independently in your the home.

For a more secure environment for living, consult the Parkinson's medical staff about certain precautions. The occupational therapist can offer ways to create a more Parkinson's friendly living space. The specialist examines items like the arrangement of furniture, handrails or toilets, as well as flooring to determine what areas of risk could pose.

How can you feel better with Parkinson's Disease Without Taking Medication

Apart from taking medication, individuals suffering from Parkinson's disease are able to increase their overall health and wellbeing keep their body functioning in good shape and reduce their symptoms. They can also improve their lives through a myriad of methods. Exercise regularly, eating a healthy diet, staying hydrated and having enough rest are just a few of those.

However, what are alternative therapies? Yoga, for instance massage, diet supplements and a myriad of other movement methods are the subject of years of study in order to discover if they aid in the treatment of Parkinson's disease. Even though the verdict is not yet being determined on certain methods, numerous non-medical methods of treatment still hold many possibilities.

Think about the following treatments that integrate:

1. Supplements for Nutrition

It is possible that you have heard about Co-Q10, an antioxidant coenzymeQ10, may help those suffering from Parkinson's disease. It is the National Institute of Neurological Disorders and Stroke however, on its part, has halted an investigation into the efficacy of Co-Q10 in 2011, when it became apparent that the supposed benefits of prevention weren't different from placebo.

If you're considering taking a supplement to treat reasons other than this discuss it with your doctor before you do so. And don't take a break from your medication.

Calcium is one of the supplements that could prove beneficial to those suffering from Parkinson's disease because the majority of calcium-rich food items (such like dairy items) are also rich in protein. This can hinder the absorption of medication.

2. Tai Chi

Since this kind of exercise can improve stability and coordination so it is natural to suggest that it can benefit those suffering from Parkinson's disease. An investigation conducted in 2012 of three kinds of exercises -such as stretching, weight training as well as tai chishowed that tai-chi assisted people suffering from moderate Parkinson's disease increase their stability and balance.

3. Yoga

Yoga has been proven to aid those suffering from Parkinson's disease improve their balance and flexibility, and it is possible that yoga can have the similar results. According to research from 2012 it is believed that yoga could improve the strength, balance, mobility and flexibility among people who suffer from movement disorders such as Parkinson's disease. Yoga can also aid in helping to improve sleep quality and increase your mood.

4. Massage

The benefits of massage for helping to reduce the symptoms associated with Parkinson's disease, especially tremor is evident regardless of whether the treatment is lasting. An analysis of research conducted in 2016 showed that massages lasting 60 minutes reduced the tightness of muscles and reduced the tremor at rest.

5. Movement Treatments

Certain movements therapies can help combat the signs of Parkinson's illness, which can affect balance and causes the gradual decline in motor capabilities. Like using the Alexander Technique, which emphasizes the balance and posture, can help people suffering from Parkinson's disease to maintain their mobility.

It is believed that the Feldenkrais Method is another therapy which aims to train your body to do challenging moves. Although you may not practice "formal" movement treatments, exercises like dancing or strength exercise (lifting weights or using fitness equipment) could help ease certain signs. Prior to beginning a new exercise regimen, talk to your doctor.

Chapter 15: What To Know About Parkinson's Diet

Parkinson's disease is an autoimmune disease that is that is caused by a neurologic issue. Certain food habits are linked to lower chance of developing Parkinson's disease. Adjusting your diet to a certain degree can aid some people suffering from Parkinson's disease to manage the symptoms.

Anybody could be infected by the disease Parkinson's. But, it is affecting about 50% of men than it affects women.

Here are some of the most frequent Parkinson's-related symptoms:

* Shaking

* Stiffness

* Walking Difficulties

* Issues Of Balance

* Difficulties With Coordination

It is common for Parkinson's symptoms to manifest slowly, over the course of several years. An occasional tremor on one hand as well as an general feeling of muscle stiffness could be early signs.

As per the National Institutes of Health (NIH) about 50,000 individuals living in the United States are diagnosed with Parkinson's disease per year.

One thing that could reduce the chance of developing Parkinson's disease and even stop the progression of it is a healthy diet.

Parkinson's Disease-Friendly Foods

These foods may assist in slowing the progress of Parkinson's disease or lower the likelihood of getting Parkinson's disease.

* Omega-3 Fatty Acids as well as fish oil

Based on certain research the fish oil can in reducing the severity of Parkinson's disease.

Omega-3 fats were found in research studies to decrease the inflammation of nerves, improve the neurotransmission of neurons, and slow down neurodegeneration. Patients suffering from Parkinson's disease could be benefited by eating more omega-3 rich fish and using supplements to omega-3.

The following seafood and fish are rich in omega-3 fatty acids

* Mackerel

* Salmon

* Herring

* Oysters

* Sardines

* Anchovies

Omega-3 fatty acids which are plentiful in fish oil, offer numerous positive health effects. They can also assist in improving cognitive health and heart health and the reduction of cognitive decline.

Omega-3 fatty acids could aid in reducing the likelihood of confusion and dementia generally as well as giving immediate benefits to those who suffer from Parkinson's disease. They are also signs of Parkinson's disease.

Beans fava

Levodopa is one of the most efficient Parkinson's treatment for Parkinson's. Since fava beans are rich in levodopa and other nutrients, people have the impression that they could help alleviate the signs of Parkinson's.

The benefits of Fava beans can be beneficial to people suffering from Parkinson's disease. However it is not recommended to use them as a substitute for prescription drugs.

There isn't much study regarding the efficacy of fava beans for reducing the development of Parkinson's disease. One study indicates that consuming fava beans may assist people with Parkinson's disease increase their ability to move and without causing any adverse unwanted side effects.

Foods Rich In Nutrients That People May Be Lacking

According to a research studies, people suffering from Parkinson's disease are often suffering from nutritional deficiency, including iron Vitamin B1, vitamin C zinc, as well as vitamin D.

According to the study the impairments could be related to neuroinflammation as well as neurodegeneration. Both are key factors in the development of Parkinson's disease.

Therefore, individuals who suffer from Parkinson's disease might opt to consume greater amounts of the food items as listed below.

Iron-Containing Foods

Iron is present in the following food items:

* Liver

* Red Meat

* Beans

* Nuts

Vitamin B1-containing foods

Vitamin B1 is present in the following food items:

* Peas

* Bananas

* Oranges

* Nuts

* Whole Wheat Bread

Vitamin C fortified foods

Vitamin C is present in the following food items:

* Lemons And Limes

* Peppers

* Strawberries

* Broccoli

* Potatoes

Zinc-containing foods

Zinc is present in these food items:

* Meat

* Shellfish

* Bread

* Wheat Germ And Other Cereal Items

Vitamin D-fortified food items

Vitamin D is present in the following food items:

* Fatty Fish

* Red Meat

* Yolks Of Eggs

* Certain Fortified Foods

Chapter 16: Antioxidant-Containing Foods

The body's free radicals are chemical substances that can become unstable. They are necessary for a healthy well-being. But, if there's unbalance and you have higher levels of free radicals than is necessary, body's fatty tissue, DNA, as well as proteins may be affected.

Oxidative stress refers to the process to describe the harm that free radicals cause. This condition occurs when the body's concentration of free radicals becomes excessive, leading to cells to be damaged. The stress of oxidative is linked with the progression of Parkinson's disease in a number of research studies.

Antioxidants help keep the free radicals in check Thus, eating a high antioxidant diet is a good way to avoid the effects of oxidative stress. In turn, a person who suffers from Parkinson's disease could opt to incorporate antioxidant-rich food items into their diet.

Antioxidants are found in the following food items:

*Blueberries, cranberries cherries, grapes as well as raspberries are a few of the top fruits.

* Brazil nuts, pecans and walnuts

* other spices, including turmeric

* parsley-like herbs such as rosemary

* cacao and cocoa powder

* Artichokes, broccoli spinach and Kale

* limes and lemons

* tea verde

* navy beans, kidney beans beans, as well as black beans

In General, A Healthy Diet

Although the above-mentioned foods might be helpful to those who suffer from Parkinson's disease essential that they focus on the overall nutrition of their diet.

Be sure to follow these nutritional guidelines:

Beware of fad diets, and take the time to consume the right foods in every category.

There should be plenty of grain, vegetables and fruit should be eaten.

Use sugar with moderation.

Limit your sodium and salt consumption.

The foods that contain antioxidants, such as vividly colored, dark fruit as well as vegetables, are best eaten.

Follow a low-fat and low-saturated fat and a low-cholesterol diet.

Be sure to drink alcohol in moderation.

Beware of these food items.

There is a myriad of foods that could exacerbate signs of the disease, or accelerate its progress. Here are a few of these.

Foods processed for processing

Certain studies indicate that the "Western-style" diet is associated with increasing the severity of Parkinson's disease.

Foods processed are abundant within this diet. These processed foods comprise the following:

Foods In Cans

Sodas

Cereals For Breakfast

Chips

Bacon

Ready-To-Eat Meals

Candy

Cakes

Based on one research, many of these food items including canned foods as well as sodas, can be linked in "rapid [Parkinson's] progression."

Furthermore, consuming lots of processed food "contributes to increased intestinal permeability and dysbiosis due to an excess of gram-negative bacteria," as per the study's author of a separate study.

They further say that intestinal permeability is more likely to be associated with an "positive connection" with the intensity of Parkinson's disease.

It could be because of the neurotoxic chemicals emitted by the bacteria that enter the bloodstream, causing gut-related symptoms, which spread to the oropharynx (food pipe) and the oral cavity as per the study.

Parkinson's disease manifests itself in signs such as difficulty swallowing, talking, as well as smell.

Patients with Parkinson's disease might prefer to stay away from processed foods as they may be associated with an increase in symptom severity.

Some Dairy Products

Based on a variety of research, dairy products have been associated with an increased chance of developing Parkinson's disease. For instance, one study indicates that the consumption of low fat and skim milk could increase the chance of getting this disease.

A different study indicates the consumption of cheese and yogurt can speed up the progression of Parkinson's disease.

Therefore, a person who suffers from Parkinson's disease could be advised to limit their consumption of large quantities of dairy items.

Saturated fat and cholesterol-containing foods

In accordance with several studies that have been conducted, eating a lot of fat may increase the risk of developing Parkinson's disease.

While a greater intake of cholesterol increases the likelihood of developing Parkinson's disease. However, a more frequent intake of polyunsaturated fat acids will reduce the likelihood of getting.

In the end the sufferer of Parkinson's disease could need to reduce the amount of cholesterol they consume to help in reducing the symptoms. Additionally, they may want to reduce the amount of saturated fats that are present in their food.

But, further research on the relationship between diet and fat and Parkinson's diseases is necessary.

Difficult-To-Chew Foods

The swallowing and chewing process is a challenge for a lot of people suffering from Parkinson's disease. If this happens it is necessary to seek medical attention. Speech and language therapy could be able to help with this issue.

But, if someone has difficulty chewing and swallow certain foods it is best to avoid them.

The most common of them can be found:

Tough Foods

Crumbly, Dry Foods

Foods That Are Rough Or Chewy

If someone insists on eating chewy food They can make sauces or gravy to soften them, making easier to eat.

It is also possible to make the it more soft by cutting it into smaller pieces or placing it in casseroles.

Consuming a drink with meals can aid in chewing and swallowing.

Summary

The next most common neurodegenerative disease is Parkinson's. Stiffness, shakes as well as difficulty walking and balance are some of the symptoms. People with Parkinson's disease may struggle with coordination.

There is a wide variety of food items that are able to assist people suffering from Parkinson's symptoms. Fava beans, fish oils as well as antioxidant-rich foods, food items high in vitamin B1, C, and D are a few of them.

People suffering from Parkinson's disease could also need to steer clear of certain foods. Foods that are processed, such as canned fruits as well as vegetables, and dairy items like yogurt, cheese and milk with low fat and food items that are high in cholesterol and saturated fats fall in the category of saturated fat and cholesterol.

The problems of swallowing and chewing can be common for people with Parkinson's disease. Therefore, food items which are hard to swallow or chew including tougher foods, can be kept away from.

Chapter 17: Parkinson's Disease Natural Treatments

A lot of people don't know about alternatives to non-pharmaceutical the treatment of Parkinson's disease. There are many organic supplements and medications to help manage the symptoms of Parkinson's disease. They can also assist with the terrible side effects Parkinson's medications can trigger. It's crucial to look into these alternatives to determine which one best suits your needs.

Vitamin-D

Vitamin D is vital in brain and nerve functioning in addition to managing mood. Vitamin D levels have been associated to depression according to studies, and taking supplements with vitamin D supplements can help ease this condition. Depression is among the more common symptoms that are not motor of Parkinson's disease. It affects nearly half of the people with the condition.

Magnesium L-Threonate and Magnesium

As well as despair, those who suffer from Parkinson's disease typically have anxiety throughout their disease. The anxiety isn't linked with progress in the disease, but it could occur prior to or following an PD diagnosis and often coexists with depression. As high as 50% of patients with Parkinson's may experience feelings of sadness or anxiety at times during their treatment.

Magnesium is a vital food mineral that is also the second-most frequent electrolyte. Magnesium deficiencies are commonplace within the Western diet, and has been linked to various negative adverse health effects, such as an anxiety, cramps, weakness as well as high blood pressure. Magnesium deficiencies have also been linked to Alzheimer's disease type 2 diabetes, as well as heart disease.

An extensive review that was published in 2017 reviewed the results of 18 different research studies. The study found that magnesium supplements may help people with anxiety, but further evidence is required for this particular area. It is advised that people seeking magnesium supplements for anxiety, start by taking a small dosage, like 100 mg. Do do not exceed 350 mg per day, without consulting with a physician.

Both genders should consume 400-420 mg or 320-360 mg each day, according to the age of the person, in order to alleviate different symptoms associated with Parkinson's disease, including fatigue as well as muscle cramps and weakness as well as constipation. Magnesium can be toxic and cause diarrhoea.

Magnesium L'Threonate is a specific Magnesium which we recommend for people suffering from Parkinson's disease. There are a variety of supplements of Magnesium that may help alleviate the symptoms of Parkinson's disease, however Magnesium L-Threonate is unique due to studies that have proven that this kind of magnesium can assist in improving memory as well as general cognitive functioning. Magnesium L-

Threonate is demonstrated to aid in recall, learning as well as cognitive wellbeing in various studies.

Magnesium L'Threonate is a top-quality magnesium supplement that was developed by MIT researchers (MIT is a private research institute located situated in Cambridge, Massachusetts). It's the sole type of magnesium proven to deliver magnesium-rich elements directly to the brain. Furthermore, it's associated with various cognitive advantages as well as the standard magnesium-related benefits.

Vitamin B

B vitamins comprise of eight essential nutrients which are used in conjunction to manage a wide range of bodily functions, such as high levels of stress. Vitamin B12 deficiency could lead to a myriad of neurological signs including nerve damage, neuropathy and impairment of cognitive function. In a study conducted in 2017 of those suffering from the lowest levels of vitamin B-12 in their bloodstream are more prone to be afflicted by stress or sadness. Foods high with B vitamins, like yogurt-based spreads, such as Marmite and Vegemite were less anxious and levels of stress than people who didn't as per a study from 2018. study. This was the case especially for spreads that contained vitamin B12. The research conducted previously has revealed that people with low B12 levels experience a quicker development in PD symptoms than people with more levels. The research suggests that stopping or rectifying bad B12 levels early may delay the progression of the disability that is associated with Parkinson's disease.

L-theanine

Black and green teas contain L-theanine which is an amino acid. It could be a mild anxiolytic and sedative, in accordance with some studies. Drinkers who consumed a drink that contained 200 mg of l-theanine experienced lower stress-related responses as well as cortisol levels following an activity that was difficult than who consumed a placebo drink, in a double-blind trial. Start with the most effective dosage of l-theanine is suggested. These supplements typically come in 200 mg tablets. The recommended dosage is no greater than 400 mg, without consulting a physician before taking it.

Omega-3 acid fatty acids

They are present in fish-based meals as well as flaxseed. Based on the Office of Dietary Supplements they play an important role for brain health. As the body can't make these fats, we require them from foods. A meta-analysis and systematic review that was published in the year 2018 reviewed the results of 19 studies conducted in clinical settings and concluded that using an omega-3 supplement such as fish oil may help people suffering from anxiety. In a review from 2018 study, low intake of omega-3 fats can raise the chance of developing anxiety or depression. Therefore, taking omega-3 supplements may help to prevent or alleviate these signs.

CBD

CBD is a natural chemical in the cannabis plant. Cannabinoids are the term used to describe these chemical compounds. There are a myriad of these substances found in cannabis, however just a handful of them are known and researched. CBD isn't intoxicating as the other components of the tetrahydrocannabinol (THC) that is the most known cannabinoid from cannabis. However, it does possess some advantages that could be beneficial. CBD has been demonstrated in research studies to aid in relieving pain, anxiety as well as neuroprotection.

Tremors and CBD

The most well-known Parkinson's treatments can cause the tremors to become uncontrollable or even a flurry of muscle. Therapy with this drug may be ineffective --

actually, it could increase the severity of symptoms.

A previous, less extensive study showed that CBD may help ease the muscle spasms as an effective solution.

For Sleep CBD

For people suffering from Parkinson's disease and sleep disturbance, as well as a deficiency in high-quality sleep is a major concern. There is a common occurrence of vivid nightmares or dreams, and also to experience movement while you sleep.

Both CBD and cannabis may help with sleep issues According to research.

Life Expectancy

Researchers have suggested that CBD can help improve the living quality for people suffering from Parkinson's disease due to the numerous benefits it could bring. People suffering from Parkinson's disease need to be worried about this.

CBD intake improved the quality of life for people suffering from Parkinson's disease, who were not suffering from psychiatric or neurological illnesses, as per one study. Since this research involved an insignificant sample of people further research is required in order to verify the results.

Pruriens Mucuna (velvet bean)

Mucana Pruriens is the name of a leguminous species which has been utilized for centuries in Ayurvedic therapy to treat Parkinson's disease over the years. It grows in the wild in subtropical and tropical regions around the world has seeds high in levodopa, as well as two other components of mitochondrial electron transport chain, namely coenzyme Q10 as well as nicotine adenine dinucleotide (NADH). The mucuna seed-based powder showed comparable efficacy as levodopa when it comes to reducing Parkinsonian symptoms using a single dose randomized controlled study. As compared to levodopa formulation showed a quicker start and resulted in fewer dyskinesias.

In yet another study In a different study, Mucuna Puriens has been shown to be superior to levodopa/benserazide for every safety and efficacy criterion. Additionally, it was discovered that the effect of Mucuna Puriens is comparable to results of a pharmaceutical formulation of levodopa by itself at the same doses with less adverse negative effects. There are many people who use Mucuna Puriens in the present, and could provide a viable alternative for the long term to the levodopa that is available in commercially-available form.

Supplements that contain mucuna-pruriens are readily available. It's not recommended that Mucuna as well as levodopa should be used in conjunction, as they share a similar impact. If you're currently taking levodopa, and would like to try Mucuna, speak to your physician about decreasing the dosage of your medication before you begin using Mucuna.

Probiotics

Small intestinal bacteria overgrowth (SIBO) is a condition where the intestine's small is overflowing with bacteria (defined as 100-1,000 times higher than the typical quantity). SIBO is a condition that can cause symptoms like constipation, abdominal pain or diarrhoea that is recurrent, as well as the loss of weight. The condition is more frequent among people who suffer from PD and is less common in all people, based on research. It is also linked to increased motor disturbances in those suffering from PD. Probiotics can assist in treating SIBO in restoring a regular bacterial ecosystem.

Q10 is a coenzyme

Coenzyme Q10 (CoQ10) is an antioxidant which your body produces naturally. The cells in your body use CoQ10 to maintain and grow

However, as you get old the body's CoQ10 levels diminish.

CoQ10 levels have been discovered to be lower in those suffering from Parkinson's disease, heart disease and who are taking statins. Statins are medicines that lower cholesterol.

Fish, meat, as well as nuts are all a source of CoQ10. The amount of CoQ10 present in these foods is not enough to substantially increase CoQ10 levels within your body.

Chapter 18: The Parkinson's Disease: What Is It?

Parkinson's disease is an neurological disease that hinders a person's ability to regulate the movements of their body.

The condition usually progresses over time so that it's not obvious immediately. A slight shake within your hands could appear unimportant initially but over time, it may alter your speech, gait and sleep patterns, as well as the ability of your brain to concentrate.

If you're older than 60 then you are at a greater likelihood of developing it. Rarely, it may be diagnosed earlier.

While there's no cure for Parkinson's but therapy and help are offered to assist with the management of symptoms.

What Changes Does Parkinson's Cause In The Brain?

The substantia nerve is an area of the basal Ganglia in the deep brain. Dopamine is a neurotransmitter, which communicates with the cerebral cortex, is made by a small portion of the cells.

Dopamine is responsible for sending signals to a nerve cell which regulates movement. This is the case when you get an itchy and you need to scratch it off or you're aiming to kick a ball but require it to be kicked.

An efficient system will ensure that your body can move smoothly and with ease. When you get Parkinson's disease, the cells in your substantia nerve begin to die.

If you don't the body's levels of dopamine are likely to decrease and it won't be able to communicate as much to keep your muscles tense and under control.

It's not clear what's changed initially. As dying cells appear and you get to a threshold at which point you begin experiencing signs.

Chapter 19: Where Does It Come From?

There are many known risk factors that can cause Parkinson's disease, including exposure to pesticides, most commonly accepted causes for Parkinson's disease are those that come from genetic.

Idiopathic Parkinson's Disease is the medical term used to describe instances that are not traceable back to a specific family. This means that they do not know the exact reason for why this happens.

There are a variety of disorders that appear to mimic Parkinson's disease, but they are in fact parkinsonism (a word used to describe Parkinson's disease-like symptoms) that are caused due to something similar to the use of certain medications for psychiatric disorders.

Parkinson's Disease In The Family

If you have a parent suffering from Parkinson's disease, it raises the risk of getting the disease, and it's likely to transmit the condition to children. But, it's only a just a little over 10% of cases.

Seven genes or more are being investigated by scientists for the development of Parkinson's disease.

The researchers have linked three of them to the early onset of the disease (meaning that the disease is present earlier than average age) (meaning that they are younger than normal age). Sometimes, changes in genes result in distinct new characteristics.

Parkinson's Disease With No Known Reason

The majority of experts believe that idiopathic Parkinson's illness is due to problems with the process your body uses to make an amino acid called A-synuclein (alpha Sy-nu-clee in) (alpha si-nu-clee-in).

Proteins are macromolecules that have an exceptionally ordered arrangement. It is a problem known as misfolding of proteins that stops your body from utilizing and breaking down some proteins.

Without a suitable outlet, proteins build up in abnormal ways, or in cells (tangles or clumps) of these proteins are known as Lewy body).

When they build up, Lewy body parts are poisonous and could cause the death of cells however this isn't true for any genetic form of Parkinson's disease.

Huntington's Disease, Alzheimer's Disease as well as other amyloidoses as well as many other amyloidoses have a similar aspect: protein misfolding.

Caused Parkinsonism

Experts have found associations with certain diseases and parkinsonism.

While these do not have the hallmarks of Parkinson's disease but they do share a number of signs and symptoms that are common to the disease and doctors might be able to consider them in making an assessment.

Some possible reasons include:

* Medications. Certain drugs possess the ability to replicate the signs of Parkinson's disease.

If you cease using the medication that's creating the Parkinson's-like symptoms before they turn permanent, symptoms should be gone. The effects that follow might persist for some time following the cessation of having the drug.

* Encephalitis. It is possible that Parkinsonism could be caused by encephalitis or inflammation in the brain.

* Other toxins and poisons. Parkinsonism may be result of breathing in pollutants such as carbon monoxide or fumes produced by welding, and even insecticides.

The cost of injuries, for instance. Brain damage can be caused by frequent blows to the head, like injuries sustained from high-impact contact sports such as boxing, hockey, football, etc. This is known by the term "post-traumatic parkinsonism."

What Is The Likelihood Of Its Spreading?

The disease of Parkinson's isn't contagious It isn't contagious, so you cannot contract it from another.

Risk factors

The factors that can increase the chances of getting Parkinson's disease include:

* Age. Parkinson's disease isn't common for young adults. As you get older, the risk increases and, consequently, it doesn't show up until late or middle the life span. The median age when an individual is diagnosed with the disease is around 60.

* Heredity. A close family member is suffering from Parkinson's disease can increase your chances of getting the disorder.

However, unless an abundance of closely related family members who suffer from Parkinson's disease, your odds of getting the disease are very minimal.

* Sex. The rate of Parkinson's disease among men is much higher than for women.

Contact with toxic substances. Experimenting with herbicides or pesticides for a long time could increase the chance of developing Parkinson's disease.

Chapter 20: What Signs Should I Look For?

Reflexions and muscle tremors are typical indicators of Parkinson's. The experts used to believe that the primary signs of Parkinson's disease were related to muscle control however, this is no longer considered to be the situation.

Symptoms Associated With Movement

"Movement-related" symptoms (sometimes called "motor" symptoms) include those afflicted by Parkinson's disease:

The patient experienced a decrease in the action (bradykinesia). This sign is essential to diagnose Parkinson's disease.

People who suffer from this disorder frequently complain of feeling weak on their muscles. But this could be a consequence of muscle control issues and not a complete decrease in strength.

* Releasing trembling that happens when muscles sit inactive. This is manifested by uncontrollable, repeated trembling of muscles, even when they're not active, and happens in approximately 80percent of those suffering from Parkinson's disease.

Essential tremors on the opposite, generally happen when muscles are resting Therefore, they're distinct from resting the tremors.

* Rigidity or stiffness. Parkinson's disease manifests as the stiffness which reminds of a lead pipe, or a cogwheel. A rigidity that is not altered no matter how much you move part of your body, is known as "lead-pipe rigidity." A combination of tremor as well as lead pipe rigidity creates cogwheel rigidity.

The name is derived from the sudden beginnings and ends of the movement (think about it like the 2nd hands on the mechanical clock).

* Stability problems in your stride or posture.

The upright posture of those suffering from Parkinson's disease is due to the disease's effects slowing down on movements and its triggering of stiffness. The symptoms typically manifest when the condition progresses.

The shorter, more shuffled stride as well as less arm movement are visible signs of the problem. Certain turns while walking could require more than one step to be completed.

The fact that you blink less often than usual is a different motor signal. A lack of control over one's facial muscles can manifest itself this manner too.

* A writing style that is cramped, or extremely tiny. A lack of muscle control can cause this condition, also known as micrographia.

* Drooling. Another sign that is caused by an affliction of facial muscles.

A mask-like appearance on the face. The signs of hypomimia are little or no expression change in the face.

Trouble eating (dysphagia). The muscles in the throat decreases the throat muscles, it can cause. Chest infections and pneumonia are more likely to happen.

The voice is not normally gentle when it talks (hypophonia). An impairment in control of the muscles in the throat and chest can cause this.

Non-Movement-Related Symptoms

It is possible that there are other signs that do not have anything related to muscle control or mobility.

These symptoms, which were not motor-related, were thought to be a sign of the illness and ought to be sought out prior to the appearance of the symptoms of motor.

Research, however, indicates that the signs could exist in the early phases of the illness. It is possible that the symptoms might be an indicators of early warning signs that begin several years, or perhaps decades prior to when signs of motor dysfunction appear.

Anomic nervous system signs can be a motor-related symptoms (with the possibility of early alert signs being that are highlighted).

Constipation and stomach issues as well as urinary incontinence the erectile disorder are just some instances of this. Hypotension orthostatic (low blood pressure while standing) is another.

* Depression.

Loss of or dysfunction in the nose (anosmia).

* Sleep disorders, such as REM sleep disorder and restless legs syndrome and periodic motion disorder of the limbs.

* Unability to focus (dementia due to the disease Parkinson's).

Chapter 21: The Parkinson's Disease Progression

The devastating effects of Parkinson's illness may not be apparent for a number of years.

The process of identifying the condition is not as efficient than knowing the way it affects each individual's daily life, and then treating them accordingly This is why the system has been abandoned.

The MDS-UPDRS is an extensive assessment tool which examines four factors that affect the quality of life you have when suffering from Parkinson's disease.

Let's begin by talking about non-motor aspects of everyday life. These are the symptoms that don't involve movement in this article, including mental impairments, mood issues, anxiety and more.

Also, it inquires whether the patient has any pain, bladder obstruction, urinary incontinence fatigue, or any other symptoms.

In the next section, we'll concentrate on the physical aspects of daily routine activities. What effects do these have on the activities or abilities that require movement are described in this article. If you are prone to the tremors that you experience, it could affect the ability of you to communicate with others, chew food and swallow it or bathe and dress and much more.

*Motor skills testing -- Section 3. This test is utilized by a physician to evaluate the physical symptoms of Parkinson's disease. These criteria are the changes in face expression, stride, the speed of walking, balance, movements speed, tremors as well as other signs of general health.

Complications with movement. Section four. In this section, a medical professional examines how Parkinson's symptoms interfere with your everyday life. It's crucial to determine the length of time you've experienced symptoms and how they've affected the way you live your life.

Reasons To Visit The Doctor

It's important to visit an expert if you are experiencing any symptoms of Parkinson's disease, in order to determine if you have diagnosed and determine if there are other cause.

When To See The Doctor And What To Anticipate

Expect to be asked lots of questions from your physician. If you're prepared with the answers and have time to explain anything that requires it. Some of the questions that your physician might be asking are: When did you notice your first signs?

*If the symptoms continue or fade at various time points?

Do you notice any changes with your conditions?

Are there triggers which make your symptoms intense?

Diagnosis

It isn't possible to be identified with only one blood or urine sample.

For an accurate diagnosis of Parkinson's disease Your neurology specialist examines your medical history, look at the symptoms you are experiencing, and perform an examination of your body and neurological system.

Dopamine transporter scans are subset of SPECT scans doctors may suggest (DaTscan). The symptoms and neurological examination is the most important factor in the diagnosis of Parkinson's disease. However these scans can aid in proving the idea that you suffer from the condition. Many people are with no issues without having the DaTscan.

To rule out any other possible causes for the symptoms you are experiencing, your doctor could conduct lab tests (such such as tests of blood).

* Imaging techniques such as MRIs and brain ultrasounds PET scans, and MRIs are able to

assist in the diagnosis of other conditions in addition. The disease of Parkinson's is a notoriously challenging to identify using imaging methods.

*Carbidopa levodopa (Rytary, Sinemet, others) is a drug combination for the treatment of Parkinson's disease. It can be prescribed by your physician as a supplement to an exam.

A small dose for two days won't provide any evidence, so it is necessary to receive lots of doses to experience the results. Most of the time, a positive reaction to the drug can be used as a conclusive proof that you are indeed suffering with Parkinson's disease.

Chapter 22: Complications

Additional, possibly curable conditions are frequently associated with Parkinson's disease:

Mental stress is a major cause of. There is a possibility that you are suffering from cognitive problems (dementia) or the fatigue of your mind. These symptoms are prevalent in people suffering from advanced Parkinson's disease. The use of medication is not always helpful with the cognitive problems that cause these.

Depression and mood swings There is a chance that you'll experience the first signs of depression. The treatment for depression may improve the your quality of life as well as reduce the severity of Parkinson's disease.

The changes in your emotional state including anxiety anger, anxiety, or loss of motivation is also a possibility. The doctor can prescribe medications to treat these symptoms.

• Trouble swallowing. As your health deteriorates and you get older, you might have problems swallowing. It is possible to snore if you are having trouble swallowing, and saliva is accumulating inside your mouth.

It is difficult to chew and swallow. When the problem gets worse, it can affect the muscles of the mouth, causing it to become more difficult to chew. This can lead to the mouth to become malnourished and choke.

• Sleep disruption as well as other sleep-related problems. Patients with Parkinson's disease usually have sleep issues, for example awakening multiple times throughout the night, waking up early in the morning or falling asleep off throughout the day.

Sleeping in a coma is an indication of a rapid eye movements that are a sign of sleep disorders. It is possible to take a medication to treat your sleepiness.

*Urinary tract ailments. Bladder problems, like problems with urination or incontinence are associated with Parkinson's disease.

* Constipation. The Parkinson's disease can be linked to an inefficient digestive system that can cause constipation in the majority of sufferers.

In addition, you might feel:

There are changes of blood pressure. If your blood pressure falls quickly as you stand up and you feel it, you could experience signs such as lightheadedness, dizziness, or dizziness (orthostatic hypotension).

The smell is a problem. The ability to smell is impaired. Certain smells, or distinct smells that exist, could seem unfamiliar to you.

* Fatigue. Later in the day, fatigue and loss of energy is a common occurrence for people suffering from Parkinson's disease. However, sometimes it's not clear where the source of the issue can be identified.

* Pain. The symptom of pain is common of people suffering from Parkinson's disease. The condition is either localized or general.

Disruptions in sexual function. An increase in sexual desire or performance could be observed by people suffering from Parkinson's disease.

Prevention

Uncertain of the triggers that cause Parkinson's disease, efficient preventative actions are also difficult.

Aerobic exercise may reduce the risk of developing Parkinson's disease.

Caffeine is a chemical included in tea, coffee and even cola, was connected to a reduced chance of developing Parkinson's disease in a limited but substantial number of studies.

In addition, drinking green tea has been connected to a decrease in the likelihood of developing Parkinson's disease.

It is uncertain if coffee acts as a deterrent to the development of Parkinson's, or if there's another connection between both. As of now, there is not enough data to justify the idea that drinks containing caffeine provide protection from Parkinson's disease.

Chapter 23: Is There A Cure, And If So, What Treatment Options Are Available?

In spite of the absence of a cure, symptoms associated with Parkinson's disease can be addressed with a variety of methods.

Treatments can also vary between patients based upon symptoms and the responses to treatments. The mainstay is medication. treatment for this condition.

Implantation of a device to provide small amounts of electrical stimulation to a particular area of the brain can be a viable treatment alternative (this is also known as deep brain stimulation).

Certain people with Parkinson's disease are able to access treatment options that are experimental, including stem cells-based treatments, but the availability of these treatments varies greatly.

Medications

If you're experiencing difficulty movements, walking, or tremors, medications may assist.

Dopamine levels are increased or substituted by these medications.

The levels of dopamine within the brain are usually very low among people who suffer from Parkinson's illness. However, since it's not able to penetrate the blood-brain junction, dopamine can't be given directly.

The first time you begin treatment for Parkinson's disease can lead to a significant improvement in the symptoms.

As time passes the advantages of medication generally diminish or appear less reliable. In the majority of cases you'll be able to maintain a certain degree of control over your signs.

The doctor you see may recommend medicines such as

* Carbidopa-levodopa. The brain absorbs levodopa an organic molecule and transforms it into the neurotransmitter dopamine. This makes it the most effective therapy of Parkinson's disease.

To prevent levodopa from getting transformed into dopamine before it is out of the brain, it's typically paired to Carbidopa (Lodosyn). This can help keep the symptoms of nausea and other similar ones in check.

Diazziness and nausea can be negative side reactions (orthostatic hypotension).

If you've been taking the drug levodopa for some time, while the disease was steadily increasing, you've probably observed that its efficacy has fluctuated and decreased through time ("wearing off").

Levodopa at higher doses can result in involuntary movements (dyskinesia). If you experience any of the side effects listed above discuss with your physician regarding reducing the dosage or altering your dosage regimen.

* Carbidopa-levodopa inhalation. The combination medicine inhalation carbidopa-levodopa is available now under the name Inbrija. The drug could reduce symptoms

when oral medications abruptly cease to work during the course of.

*Infusion of levodopa and carbodopa. Combining carbidopa with levodopa creates the brand name drug Duopa. However it is absorbed into the intestines via a the feeding tube.

If you have a patient with serious Parkinson's disease that show an improvement in their response to carbidopa, but experiencing significant fluctuations in the degree of responsiveness, Duopa may be an possibility. The continuous infusion of Duopa assures that both medications remain at a constant level within the bloodstream.

The tube needs to be placed surgically, however only a small operation is needed. It is possible that the tube will be snagged or a bacterial infection may develop within the area of the infusion.

Dopamine agonists. Dopamine agonists do not convert to dopamine as levodopa. They instead act inside the brain in a way like dopamine.

In comparison to levodopa their efficacy in easing the symptoms is not as. Although they are less effective, they may be combined with levodopa, which can lessen the drug's unpredictable adverse effects.

*In in addition to pramipexole (Mirapex) and the ropinirole (Requip) Rotigotine (Rotigo) can also be an agonist of dopamine (Neupro which is an injection). If you want to get immediate relief, consider injecting the dopamine antagonist Apomorphine (Apokyn) with an extremely short duration of half-life.

There's some similarity between the negative consequences of carbidopa-levodopa as well as the undesirable side effects of dopamine antagonists.

However they may result in delusions, fatigue and even compulsions such as hypersexuality, gambling, and excessive eating. Talk about any behavior changes with your doctor if discover that you're taking the medications mentioned above and it appears to have an impact.

* Methylamine Hydroxylase Inhibitors (MAO B). Safinamide and selegiline (Zelapar) as well as rasagiline (Azilect) are some examples of these drugs (Xadago). In blocking the activities of monoamine oxidease B the brain, these drugs help in preserving Dopamine levels (MAO B). This enzyme's function is to breakdown the brain's dopamine.

Selegiline's addition to levodopa therapy could slow the development of fatigue due to drugs.

MAO B inhibitors can cause unwelcome side effects like nausea, headaches, as well as sleeplessness. In some cases, hallucinations are more frequent when the drugs are combined together with carbidopa-levodopa.

www.ingramcontent.com/pod-product-compliance
Lightning Source LLC
Chambersburg PA
CBHW051727020426
42333CB00014B/1191